YOGA
Birth Method

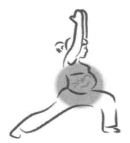

About the Author

Dorothy Guerra is a prenatal yoga teacher and a registered birth coach (doula). Owner of Birth Yoga Studio, where she runs pregnancy classes, teaches the Yoga Birth Method to couples, and trains instructors. Her method is offered as a distance-training course worldwide, certifying doulas, yoga teachers, and birth professionals. Guerra frequently speaks at conferences and hosts the television program *Get Loud about Your Life* in her home city of Toronto, Canada. She is also an advocate for women's rights for safe birth in developing countries. Volunteering in rural Kenya, providing clean safe birth kits to women with limited medical access. www.rebirththeworld.org

For more visit www.yogabirthmethod.com.

YOGA

Birth Method

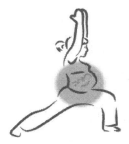

A Step-by-Step Guide for a Calm and Natural
Childbirth Experience

DOROTHY GUERRA

Yoga Birth Method Institute Publishing
Canada

second edition

Third Printing, 2018

Cover design by Fotografia Boutique
Cover woman: Maili J. Carpino   Interior illustrations by
Lynn Shwadchuk

YBM logo is owned by Dorothy Guerra and cannot be reproduced or used without instructor certification by the user. Contact the Yoga Birth Method Organization at http://yogabirthmethod.com

Library of Congress Cataloging-in-Publication Data Guerra, Dorothy.
  The yoga birth method : a step-by-step guide for natural childbirth /

  Dorothy Guerra.—First edition.
     pages cm
ISBN 978-0-9781047-2-6
  Active childbirth. 2. Natural childbirth. 3. Hatha yoga. I. Title. RG662.G84 2013
  618.4'5—dc23

Please Note

This book is a hands-on method of pain management using a natural approach with yoga techniques. If you have a high-risk pregnancy or your medical doctor has diagnosed you with a medical risk, this book may not cover those risks in detail. By using the Yoga Birth Method, you do so of your own free will and at your own risk. The author, publisher, and the Yoga Birth Method Organization assume no liability or responsibility for any complications that may arise during your pregnancy or labor.

This book is dedicated to my children, Antonio and Alessia, for teaching me the beauty in giving birth and the joy it brings forever after.

To all women who have had the joy of using yoga birthing and to all those who will.

To everyone that helped me pull this together and get it out to the world.

Maili J. Carpino for modeling her pregnancy

Maggie Habieda from Fotographia Boutique for her fabulous photography and design of the cover for this second edition

A special thanks to April Kurtyka, Sarah Townson, Danielle Downey, and Lisa Khera for sharing their Yoga Birth Method experiences in this book.

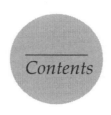

Contents

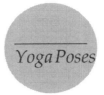

Yoga Poses

Introduction

The Yoga Birth Method (YBM) is a way to use yoga in labor to manage a natural and calm birth experience. This method is effective and powerful. It gives you motivation to stay connected to your child as you make informed decisions toward a natural birth. I will teach you how to apply yoga philosophy during your labor to remain mindful and in control of your experience, and how to incorporate the practice of postures and breathing techniques to manage progression and pain. If you have never practiced yoga, don't worry; this method is safe for everyone and can be practiced daily or as often as you wish, even before the baby arrives. The best part is that I will even teach you how to get your partner involved to encourage a daily practice and to be hands-on during the big day.

The Yoga Birth Method can be used by every woman wanting to have a positive childbirth experience no matter what her level of yoga understanding is. The techniques are simple and easy to use. If you have never taken a yoga class in your life, don't feel intimidated. Once you read through this eight-step pathway in chapter 5, you will feel comfortable using it to prepare for labor as well as using it throughout your entire labor. You may even decide to keep it up permanently after your baby is born to help you get into pre-baby shape and help you relax and enjoy your new family life.

If you have a regular practice already, this method will deepen your understanding of prenatal yoga's safe poses for pregnancy and encourage you to practice poses that are beneficial to labor. Ultimately, you will bring your practice into your labor as a way to manage your attitude, pain, and energy physically and mentally. As you read, you will notice labor is not black and white; there is no textbook description of how your labor will unfold for sure. Labor is described in a grey scale and is mostly dictated by the choices you make and the needs of your baby. All you can do for sure is be informed of all the grey matter and have an action plan to manage your mind, body, and spirit on the big day.

I assume you are reading this book because you want to birth naturally. You might even be wondering, "what is the difference between natural and medicated births?" Natural birth is when a woman goes through the entire labor without any medication administered to her body. She relies on breathing and her own birth strategy to fully complete the labor to delivery. A medicated birth is when the labor needs to be intervened by using medications to either start the labor, progress the labor, assist in pain management, or ensure the safety of mom and baby.

There are many types of medications used to help certain situations (I explain these situations in chapter 7), but it's important to know that using medication for pain does not always mean a pain-free labor. One of the main reasons women opt to avoid medications is because there are side effects, and most often these medications pass through mom's bloodstream and into the baby's. If baby does not react well to the medication, their heart rate can take a sudden turn to slower or quicker that could lead to emergency delivery. Baby also may come into this world groggy, which can affect their reaction to breastfeeding, or mom might not react well to the medication.

In any case, anytime medical drugs are introduced, there are always risks that need to be evaluated. However, my goal is to help you work through these situations and make the best decisions for you and your baby, whether you move through a fully natural birth or choose to incorporate modern medicine. In chapter 7 I describe many situations of medical intervention and teach you how to manage your choices and how the Yoga Birth Method will be an education resource for you before making any immediate intervention decisions under pressure.

If this is your first baby, you may have no idea what to expect and may already have convinced yourself you won't be able to go through it without pain medication—or, alternatively, you may be adamant that natural is how you plan to go. Making the choice to birth naturally has many benefits for you and your baby, such as the ability to move during contractions, being able to feel yourself pushing, and being able to get up and walk after birth; also, your baby will be more alert at birth and will be more likely to breastfeed easier; the list can go on and on. However, in order to truly birth naturally, you have to be prepared with a technique that will help you manage the difficulties of pain, exhaustion, and frustration. Once your labor begins, staying committed to a natural choice becomes your challenge. The practice of the Yoga Birth Method will give you the motivation and tools you need to make it possible. In chapter 5 you will be given an eight-step pathway to follow that will help you control how you move through contractions, breathe through intense pain, manage negative emotions, and ultimately control your labor from start to finish. This is your step-by-step guide for natural birth experience.

As a registered yoga teacher, registered prenatal yoga teacher, doula, and childbirth educator, I have all the tools to support your childbirth experience. Through my work as a yoga studio owner and birth coach, I was inspired to create the Yoga Birth Method. I came to realize that my prenatal teaching and childbirth work fit together perfectly. I began to incorporate the classic yoga principles with my clients to help them manage their attitude toward labor. I realized that labor can be amazing—and should be amazing. The only thing women needed was a way to make that possible, to be guided through movement and breathing and be able to increase pain tolerance as pain increased. My work with prenatal yoga helped fit this missing piece of the puzzle, and I began to give women poses and breathing techniques that matched the emotional and physiological stages of labor. Naturally, the Yoga Birth Method was born! My goal is to teach women they *CAN* take charge of *their* birth story, even within the medical system. Women can have beautiful births that are not medical processes, and they can be in full control of their birth, with the right educational tools. You can feel like you own the choices that unfold in your labor. Regardless of whether your birth is natural or medicated, it is *your* labor, and throughout this book I will empower and support you to make the right decisions for you and your baby along the way.

This is a wonderful time in your life, filled with physical changes as your body nourishes your growing baby. We will cover yoga for pregnancy in chapter 2, which will address some of these changes. The information in this book is your reliable resource for how to make it through your labor with as much ease and fearlessness as possible. I say fearlessness because I know that over the nine months of your pregnancy, you inevitably will have worries and anxiety over what labor will be like. This is normal. This book will empower you to work through anxiety and provide you the support you need to feel confident about the birthing process. I plan to demystify any negative views about the birth process you might have and help you prepare for a calm and peaceful experience based on fact, knowledge, and self-empowerment.

The reality is that giving birth to your child is as natural as grass growing on your front lawn or trees growing in a forest. Birth is a way of existence. Animals on this planet do it without ob-gyn appointments and hospitals. Women in impoverished countries do it without luxury or medical support. I am not suggesting that natural childbirth means to go it alone, without help or luxury—by all means, enjoy a wonderful environment at home or in the hospital and rely on your medical support team to assist you in a positive and resourceful way. Natural childbirth means to experience labor and birth in the most enjoyable, mindful, and unmedicated way possible, because that is how Mother Nature intended it to be.

Why would you want to experience birth naturally and feel all the pain that comes with it as opposed to being medicated and pain free?

Well, the answer is different for every woman. But for the purpose of choosing a natural birth, the answer is that *IT IS* the best way for you to be connected to your baby and in control of your body while you and your baby work together throughout the birthing process.

Using medication is a coping strategy for mom to handle and practically eliminate the intensity of pain, but what about the baby's work? When you use medication, you separate yourself from the baby in essence, you "check out" and let your baby go at it solo. Your baby must go through a series of movements that will be explained later in this book. These movements require your child to tuck and turn and fit through the birth canal. In addition, your baby undergoes a temporary change in bone structure to be able to fit their head comfortably through your pelvis. Through the entire length of your labor, your baby depends on good, strong contractions to make this process easier. When you use medication or take an epidural to early into the labor, the quality of your contractions are put at risk and your baby has a harder time working their way to the birth canal and could be the cause of a necessary C-sections.

Let me clarify that sometimes medication is necessary; if the laboring woman is experiencing major fears inhibiting labor to progress or if her panic is causing the baby to show signs of dystocia (difficulty during the birthing process), then medication may be the best option to help restore her to a calm state and get things back on track. (I discuss dystocia further in chapter 3.) The concept of the Yoga Birth Method is to prepare you for a calm state prior to labor and encourage you to start labor with mindfulness and inner peace in order to avoid possible complications for maternal and fetal distress. If you practice the techniques outlined in the eight-step pathway, you will eliminate fear and anxiety from your birth experience.

The tools in the Yoga Birth Method are designed to tackle signs of distress and empower you to embrace a connection to your child through the entire labor so that medication can be avoided. The key to choosing natural labor is to know what to expect and eliminate the fear factor. Being informed and aware of the physiological and emotional stages of labor prepares you with a coping strategy. Childbirth is considered labor because in many ways it *is* work; with this method, I will guide you through that work and make it efficient. Labor does not have to be painful and exhausting. The tools in this book will guide you through a process to help manage your perception of labor. It will also help you understand your baby's role in labor and give you the ability to work together as a team. Together you allow the experience of pain to be something you are working with and not against. These tools are specific and don't require you to figure out what option works best. It is a disciplined approach to how to move, breathe, and think in each stage of labor. All you have to do is follow the pathway in chapter 5.

This book will help you:

- understand what yoga is and how the eight-step pathway unfolds in labor

- feel comfortable using yoga during your pregnancy and in labor with or without prior yoga experience

- understand what happens in labor physically and emotionally

- understand how to use the eight-step pathway in each stage of labor

- understand the medical aspect of birthing so that you can make informed choices

- understand how yoga in pregnancy can be more meaningful than just a physical practice: it is a journey to birth

- include your partner with hands-on techniques for labor support

- understand how to explain the Yoga Birth Method so that others are equipped with the tools to have a mindfully natural birth experience

Here is a list of questions most frequently asked about the Yoga Birth Method.

What is the Yoga Birth Method?

The Yoga Birth Method is an eight-step birthing pathway that empowers women through a natural and mindful childbirth experience. YBM's philosophy is for the mother to connect with her baby during childbirth and to engage in her labor as an experience of enlightenment. A very specific sequence of breathing and postures adapted to the physical and emotional changes in the stages of labor enables women to manage contractions from a calm, meditative, and controlled perspective.

What is the purpose of the Yoga Birth Method?

The purpose of the Yoga Birth Method is to give women a greater opportunity to embrace childbirth as a natural and joyful experience. How a woman gives birth becomes her birth story, and that birth story is shared each time she reflects on the birth of her child. I founded YBM as a way to give women the best birth story possible. Yoga is an ancient practice of breathing, movement, and concentration that invokes personal well-being and stress-free living. This method applied to childbirth gives women the exact same experience during the challenges of labor.

How does it work?

There are eight steps for a woman to use. By following the eight steps, she does not need to try to manage contractions. The pathway is a natural progression of mindful awareness of birth intentions, movement that aligns the mother's pelvis to the baby's cardinal birthing movements, and breathing strategies that manage the physical exertion in the first stage of labor. When she uses the sequence in labor, it becomes a natural and effortless embodiment of meditation.

Why does it work?

It works because the mother chooses two intentions (from a list of ten) that are based on the mother's personal behavior characteristics, and these become her point of focus during birth. Her goal is to be mindful of her actions and to be consistent in managing her birth story throughout labor. The YBM sequence of postures and breathing helps her manage the challenge of contractions, and as they intensify over the stages, the sequence changes to adapt to these changing intensities. She is fully present to what is happening to her body as her baby works to be born. When she is present, she is better equipped to make the right decisions during labor and utilize her right of choice.

I have never done yoga; will this method still work for me?

Yes, because you follow a specific pathway that is simple and yet very profound in action. It does not require yoga experience, just a willingness to use the method and a determination to have a positive birth story.

What if I don't understand yoga terms?

The pathway is described in layman's terms and can be used interchangeably for those who would like to embrace the Sanskrit philosophy and for those who want the English words.

Do I need to have a partner?

The YBM can be used with or without a partner. The techniques are ultimately used by the birthing woman, and a partner can support the process.

What are the benefits of doing this method?
The benefits are:

- faster labor progression, as the postures encourage the baby's movement into the birth canal with quicker dilation and effacement
- a better chance at natural labor, as the meditative aspect allows a woman to remain focused and in control of her birth experience in a positive manner
- a deeper connection to the baby's efforts during birth
- less likelihood of medications and interventions, as the tools are specific for the mother's physical and emotional needs during each phase of labor
- the mother is present and fully aware at the moment of birth because she was able to manage a natural pathway
- the baby is fully awake and aware at birth, which may not be the case if medications are used

How does this method compare to others?
Most birthing techniques use breathing and meditation techniques. However, this method is unique because it is based on a deep connection between mother and child during birth. The mother is necessarily fully present to her experience of pain during birth—as opposed to pain happening to her—to help her baby be born into the world. There is no reference to external distraction. The meditations, or birth intentions, are directly related to her personal behavioral characteristics, and the tools to manage pain are specific and outlined.

Do I need any special training to do the method?

No. If you would like to be prepared and educated before labor begins, become acquainted with the intention selection (see chapter 1) and familiarize yourself with the sequence. However, if you would like to take a course or workshop on YBM, that is available to you, and you also have the opportunity to use a YBM-trained doula. See www.yogabirthmethod.com for more information.

Is this method safe?

Yes, this method is safe and effective for the baby and for the mother. If you have a high-risk pregnancy or have been diagnosed with Strep B, preeclampsia, gestational diabetes, placental dystocia, a breech baby, or any other risk factors, it is important you speak to your doctor about natural childbirth options no matter what birthing method you use. Here I will uncover ways in which you can still incorporate the Yoga Birth Method to help you work through these concerns.

I would like to incorporate YBM in my birthing plan, but I want the option of using medication.

Using the YBM requires an open mind to natural childbirth. If you decide that you would like medication during your labor process after applying the techniques, then you are still able to continue with the method and use the meditative and breathing tools. You may lose the ability to apply the posture sequence, as some medications such as an epidural (an anesthetic administered into the spine) require a mother to remain in bed during labor and restrict her ability to have freedom of movement.

I am planning to have my baby in the hospital. Is this method only for a natural birthing environment?

The method can be applied anywhere you choose to birth your child.

There are no certified trainers in my area.
How can I access this method?

Using a trained YBM practitioner is a personal preference. By reading this book and applying the techniques, you will receive enough information to use the method in your labor without a certified practitioner. This method outlines all the necessary techniques to begin your own YBM practice or incorporate the techniques into an already established practice. If you decide to inquire about certified practitioners, you can contact me at www.yogabirthmethod.com for the opportunity to have a YBM workshop in your area or to arrange a private session.

At what stage in my pregnancy should I learn this method?

There is no right or wrong time; however, the earlier you begin to educate yourself on the progression of labor, the more equipped you will be with resources. This method can be used from the onset of pregnancy, as the early labor sequence is a wonderful prenatal practice during the nine months, and it helps a woman's body to be receptive to a faster and easier birth. Using the method for the first time in the final weeks of pregnancy or during labor still puts you in an advantageous position to have a better birth story than not using it at all. Keep in mind that every woman is different and every labor is different. There are no set guarantees as to how long your laboring time will be. The YBM also does not prevent unexpected outcomes that may occur in labor; it is a technique that gives you the resources to be mindful of your labor and be better able to make informed decisions.

How can I get my child birthing coach
on board with this method?

It is important to choose a birthing coach that agrees with and understands your birth choices. If you feel you need to convince your birth coach to see things your way, you may not have the right coach for your needs. If your birth coach would like to learn how to use the Yoga Birth Method, they can visit www.yogabirthmethod.com for training dates.

**Is this just a trend like the yoga phenomenon,
or is this a method that I can count on?**

This is an effective birthing technique that helps woman manage natural childbirth. The practice of yoga has maintained a following for over five thousand years because it works, and the same will hold true with the Yoga Birth Method in years to come.

1

The Yoga Birth Method Overview

This method was born from my experience as a yoga specialist, doula, and childbirth educator. I have been teaching couples how to use yoga to manage pain in labor for years. I have seen the Yoga Birth Method's benefits in my client's births and all the way into postpartum recovery; I will share some real birth stories in this book. Yoga is a holistic practice that offers people a way to embrace their physical body. It wakes people up to the power of their thoughts and the energy of their spirit.

Yoga is a system, not a religion, over five thousand years old. Second-century philosopher C. E. Patanjali wrote the *Yoga Sutras*, which describe how to create harmony and reach an enlightened state. His work was written in Sanskrit, the ancient language of the East, and translated by many different authors. Yoga teachers around the world use his aphorisms to educate and teach students how to achieve enlightenment. The ultimate realization is that you contain a life-force energy called breath. The breath encompasses the power of the present moment. The breath is also your direct connection to childbirth. Without your ability to breathe, you lose your life; without the control of breath in childbirth, you lose your ability to manage pain and ultimately your connection to your birthing experience.

The practice of postures in yoga is meant to encourage your senses beyond your physical body and create freedom of movement. The body is considered a temple that holds the true self. By practicing movement, you encourage awakening to a deeper sense of being. In childbirth, freedom of movement is vital to managing a natural birth. The concept of movement in birth and movement in yoga is the same: movement allows you to work through pain and manage a deeper connection to what is happening within you. When you are able to acknowledge physical limitations and work through them, you tap into a powerful state of enlightenment.

My work as prenatal yoga specialist taught me to understand how the system of enlightenment can be applied to natural childbirth. The moment your child is born and you hold them for the first time, it is enlightenment. It's that simple. What people take a lifetime to master, you can experience in childbirth. The moment after birth, you will realize your purpose as a human being is far greater then self-fulfillment.

Enlightenment in the path of yoga leads students to believe that it is something hard to achieve. I don't believe that. I don't teach that enlightenment is a far-reaching or lifelong practice. In my philosophy, enlightenment consists of moments of grace and truth. They are realizations and accomplishments that happen when you are awake to them. You can become awake to them by acting like a yogini, someone who chooses to live by the laws of yoga principles. These principles are an important part of the YBM, and we will discuss them in the following pages. Learning these principles will provide the empowerment you need to be awake to your labor and encourage you and your birth partner to offer support to one another and be committed to natural, enlightened birth experience, regardless of how your birth unfolds.

Being a Yogini

The practice of yoga teaches you how to live effectively. There are eight aspects of a yogic lifestyle, called the limbs of yoga. The eight-limb system is a guide that encourages personal development through harmony of mind, body, and spirit. A yogini, a woman who practices yoga, follows these rules with the goal of achieving enlightenment or spiritual bliss. Here in the West, the authenticity of yoga has been lost to the concept that yoga means physical practice. When people go to a class and practice postures, they believe they are doing yoga. This is not the case at all. The practice of postures is just one limb in the entire system. It is called the *asana,* or posture, limb. To be disciplined in yoga, you must adhere to all eight limbs. The idea of prenatal yoga is to use the posture and breath energy limb to maintain a healthy body during pregnancy and to be physically ready to handle labor. The YBM identifies the eight limbs as a disciplined technique. Before I can address this technique for labor, it's important to understand the eight limbs, or rules, that you follow to ensure you stay true to the path of being a yogini. You need to have a sense of what the eight limbs are unrelated to giving birth. Having an understanding of what yoga means toward your own social values and responsibilities will help you use these tools later in labor to the best of your ability.

Let's take a look at the rules of a yogic lifestyle.

rule #1: Intent to Refrain
from Negative Behaviors (*Yamas*)

Yamas are your social responsibilities to others and are practiced by setting an intention to refrain from negative behaviors. *Yamas* are the practice of abstinence. There are five specific behaviors that are considered negative and harmful to others, and in yoga they are expressed in the positive as nonviolence, truthfulness, non-stealing, moderation, and nonpossessiveness. The positive presentation of the

Yamas reinforces the yogini way of life. To achieve peace, happiness and harmony with people and yourself, you must be mindful of these behaviors daily. The idea is that once you refrain from one of these behaviors, the rest will fall into place as a result. As you read the following *yamas*, recognize if one resonates with you more than another. I have asked you a series of questions after each one that will help you think deeper into the meaning of the intention. Jot your thoughts down on paper to help you decide which intentions will be your focus as we prepare your birth plan later in this book.

Nonviolence (Ahimsa)

Be mindful of your actions and ensure that you do not engage in harmful behavior. Refrain from physical and verbal violence that can be caused emotionally and mentally, not only toward society but toward yourself as well. Being mindful of ahimsa teaches you to manage aggression and anger. When you are upset or feel challenged, aggression might be your innate reaction as a coping strategy. Acting out with aggression leads to a domino effect of negativity and can make simple things worse. Rarely do problems get solved with anger or violence. When you experience emotions that prevent you from being mindful of ahimsa, take a moment to recognize how your emotions directly affect your outcomes. Harmful words and actions cannot be taken back. Removing aggression from your life can help you achieve positive experiences and help build stronger relationships.

- Do you feel the urge to curse and accuse when you are mad?

- When you get angry or upset, do you lash out at others?

- How can you become mindfully aware of your actions and thoughts that may lead to hurting others emotionally?

Truthfulness (Satya)

Be aware of your words and how you portray your emotions. You might say harmful things to others and show no regard for their feelings. Other times you may say things to please others but end up hurting yourself. Truthfulness means to be honest and sincere when speaking about your feelings while being mindful of your behavior and of your true intention behind your words. The energy of your words creates the environment you live in. If you constantly speak in a negative tone, then negative energy will become your best friend. You will attract negative things into your life and you will have more negativity to talk about. Practicing truthfulness is to be aware of the verbal energy that you put into your life. When you speak in a positive tone and speak with honesty, you allow good to come into your life and embrace an abundance of positive experiences that come from that.

- How do your words reflect truthfulness in your life?
- Do you think before you speak?
- Do you speak up for yourself?
- Do you intentionally try to bring others down?
- Are you respectful when you speak?
- Are you honest with yourself?

Non-Stealing (Asteya)

This does not specifically mean to refrain from stealing material possessions from others. It represents the idea of emotional energy that you might steal from others. When you put yourself in a position of needing too much attention or desiring what others have, you engage in the act of stealing energy. Practicing non-stealing is about managing your personality, finding a balance between extrovert and introvert. You have a responsibility to care for the people around you without greedily fulfilling your own needs. When you have good relationships surrounding you, those people will naturally give you what you need without you having to force it out of them. At the same time, you have to give back to those relationships and make the balance of give and take equal.

- Do you value other people's time?

- Where do you show neediness in your life?

- Are you able to manage crisis in your life without involving others?

- Are you helpful toward others?

- Do you balance managing your needs with others' needs?

Moderation (Brahmacharya)

By practicing moderation, you recognize that all things have limits. You cannot let one situation take over your entire life, and you cannot spend all your energy on one thought or desire. Everything in life has balance, and to achieve balance you must act with discipline. When you overindulge or overstimulate, you engage in self-destructive behavior. This leads to regret and disappointment when things are out of control. When you want more than you have or you want to control more than you can handle, you set yourself up for failure. Practicing moderation as a yogini means to know when things are out of balance and to find ways to cultivate centeredness.

- How can you be more disciplined in your life?

- Are you obsessive toward your emotions?

- Do you pay attention to experiencing moderation in your life?

- Do you take time to enjoy the small things in your life?

- Do you struggle to always have more?

Non-possessiveness (Aparigraha)

By letting yourself be open to experiencing and accepting love and care from others, you practice non-possessiveness. Let go of attachments to situations, possessions, and people. When you cling to something, you establish a sense of ownership. That attachment can lead to suffering and negative behavior. Things do not belong to you. They are meant to be enjoyed and shared. When you die, there is nothing that you can possess or control. Non-possessiveness is the practice of letting go of control, obsessions, and jealousy.

- What are you possessive over in your life?
- What do you spend the most energy trying to control or protect?
- Can you let go of attachments and be more open to sharing experiences in your life?

rule #2: Intent to Practice Positive Behaviors (Niyamas)

Niyamas are your personal responsibilities to your well-being. They are behaviors that reflect your attitude toward yourself. They are your observances in your daily actions that help you to value your worth and teach you to respect yourself. There are five important observances, and by being mindful of at least one, you naturally begin to follow the rest. As you read these *niyamas*, recognize if one resonates with you more, and jot it down. Again, it will help you choose the best intention when you get ready to start your pathway to labor.

Purity (Saucha)

This represents not only how you take care of yourself but how you think and feel. You need to practice cleanliness in your thoughts and in your environment. Purity means to take care of your health and feed your mind with positive energy. Purity teaches you to be mindful of toxicity in your life, whether it be negative relationships, situations, or your lifestyle in general. Purity teaches you respect for your body, mind, and spirit. You are a channel of energy, and everything you do reflects the energy you put out and receive. Being mindful of purity gives you the ability to keep your flow of energy positive and vibrant.

- What do you need to detoxify out of your life?
- Have you maintained a healthy lifestyle?
- Do you value what you think?
- Are you comfortable with how you look?

Contentment (Samtosha)

Being aware of what you have and where you are in your life and appreciating it is living with contentment. Be in the moment and acknowledge everything as it is, without change. Respect your life and accept everything that you are going through as a means to understand your journey. Contentment teaches you to be in the here and now and to accept circumstances as they are. When you are present, you are better able to manage your life in a direction that is rewarding. You are better able to handle difficult situations and face challenges from a calm, mindful perspective.

- Do you appreciate everything in your life?
- Are you present in each moment?
- Can you be grateful for everything you experience as is?

Discipline (Tapas)

To practice discipline, show a commitment to something. Be aware of what you want in your life, and do what it takes to achieve it with good effort. Discipline teaches you to value what you desire so that you can make an honest effort in seeing it through as a commitment to yourself. If you are faced with an obstacle or a roadblock, it is easy to give up or set limitations to your beliefs in what you think you deserve. Difficulties and challenges are part of life. They are meant to teach you to value your efforts and appreciate what you achieve. If everything was easy, there would be no joy or appreciation in life. When you are working toward a goal—no matter how simple, small, big, or overzealous—it is up to you to commit to it and to keep reminding yourself to value what you want to achieve. When things get in the way, make disciplined decisions that keep you committed.

- Do you have goals in your life?

- Do you have the willpower to accomplish your goals?

- How do you commit to seeing things through in your life?

- Do you get upset with yourself when you don't follow through?

Self-Study (Svadhyaya)

You should be able to see all things in your life as lessons. You have the ability to learn from your mistakes and to make informed choices going forward. By self-study, you learn how to manage pain, suffering, and unhappiness by knowing how you react to things and changing your behavior as a result. Practicing self-study means to awaken to your experiences and to not let things pass you by. Everything you do has meaning, even the littlest things. Be mindful of the choices you make and how they affect who you are. Know who you are and how you got to where you are. If you learn from yourself, going forward you can take steps that change your life and will bring a greater sense of joy and fulfillment.

- How do you react to difficult situations?

- Are you aware of your choices and how they affect your outcomes in daily life?

- Do you value yourself?

- How do you see yourself in someone else's eyes?

Divine Empowerment (Ishvara Pranidhana)

Surrender to something greater. Trust yourself and let go of energy that isolates you into a physical being. You have a higher purpose. You can open up to positive experiences just by opening up to the idea that all things are a gift from something far greater than you. There is purpose in all things through your process of life. There are many different religions to follow if religion represents divinity to you. Yoga is not a religion; it is a discipline. Divinity is different to all people. This is a personal struggle for some, and for others it is a strong value in their lives. Just recognizing that there is a divine energy that exists within you is part of your discovery on a yogic pathway. How you embrace it is your journey.

- Do you believe in something greater than your physical realm?
- Can you surrender to a higher power?
- Are you open to divine purpose and energy?

rule #3: Postures (*Asanas*)

Keeping your body healthy allows you to maintain physical freedom. You should be aware of your physical challenges and limitations and work toward making yourself stronger and pain-free. Your body is your connection to the physical world. Postures teach you to understand your physical health and well-being. By being mindful of your body, you have a better chance of fighting disease, illness, and injury. Posture work keeps the muscles free from tension, toxicity, and stress. When you are free from this kind of pain, you have more energy to focus on your inner spirit.

Postures in yoga are physical positions that allow the body to stretch and strengthen. They can restore the body to good health or help manage discomfort. Postures can flow to help create mobility and endurance, or they can be held to encourage flexibility and strength. Postures not only work the physical body, they also stimulate the nervous system and restore emotional well-being. By understanding the benefit to each pose, you can open and create space physically and emotionally. By being dedicated to posture work, you show respect for your body and teach yourself how to stay pain-free and in optimal shape. Postures are safe for all trimesters of pregnancy. They help you manage physical changes and encourage you to connect with your unborn child. We will cover some aspects to prenatal yoga later in this book. The YBM uses specific *asanas* in each stage of labor to encourage labor progression.

rule #4: Breath Energy (*Pranayama*)

Breath energy is awareness of breath. In yoga practice, breath is called *prana*; it is considered life-force energy. Without breath, there would be no ability to live. Each inhalation and exhalation is vital to existence and can teach you how to value the present moment. Breathing is a process that rejuvenates the cardiovascular system and stimulates your central nervous system. By inviting a calm breath into the body, you are able to control stress and how you react to it. There are many different breathing techniques in the yoga system, and each breathing technique is designed to stimulate the body and mind in a different way.

The yoga system uses breath energy combined with postures to move and build presence and awareness physically and mentally. Practicing the two in union is regarded as the highest form of self-discipline. In the YBM, we use specific breathing techniques for each phase of labor.

rule #5: Sense Withdrawal (*Pratyahara*)

Sense withdrawal means to surrender to your physical and emotional feelings, to try not to control them but to accept them and be present to them. When you are mindful of your senses, you learn to surrender to your experiences and not judge them. Things can happen, and you let them go. Live without attaching to outcomes.

This concept means to withdraw from sensory stimulations that form your thoughts and perceptions. You need to depend less on your sense of taste, touch, smell, touch, and sight and more on your inner ability to accept what is. When you fuel your emotions with external pleasures, you create a false sense of reality. Your ability to experience and understand things should come from within. To fully withdraw means to surrender to action without judgment and live without expectation. The YBM uses sense withdrawal as a way to experience the act of giving birth without attaching to the physical sense of pain.

rule #6: Mindfulness (*Dharana*)

Mindfulness is concentrating on one thing without distraction. By practicing mindfulness, you learn to limit the fluctuations of the mind and become focused. You eliminate all other thoughts and teach the mind discipline. When you are able to concentrate on one task, you develop patience and determination. Mindfulness is used with *asanas* and breath energy to bring a conscious awareness to the physical body as a temple that holds who we are. Concentration techniques in yoga practice help prepare the body and mind for a deeper meditative state. *Mantras*—simple words or sentences that you can repeat over and over again—are a way to increase mind control. When you practice mantras, you repeat positive words or sentences that replace mind chatter. Mantras create space in your thoughts that releases negativity and distraction. In the YBM, mindfulness is an integral part to managing the entire labor experience. You will learn forty mantras in chapter 2 that you can use in labor.

rule #7: Meditation (*Dhyana*)

Meditation is the practice of complete disassociation of body and thought. It refers to taking the body into a state where you can experience an essence of complete freedom physically and emotionally. When you reach this state, you become aware of a deeper energy that releases you from pain and suffering. Meditation is practiced in different ways: lying down, sitting, or from practicing deep concentration in postures. Meditating can be difficult and requires discipline. The difficulty with meditation is that people try to jump right into it. In order to meditate effectively, there has to be a preparation for silence and stillness. Meditation can be practiced in every moment of your day. By learning how to be mindful of negative and positive behaviors, keeping the body tension-free to sit through meditation, breathing with presence, and practicing concentration, you ease into a meditative state that is natural. The YBM teaches you to experience meditation as a calm state through each stage of labor.

rule #8: Enlightenment (*Samadhi*)

Enlightenment is the ultimate goal of practicing yoga. When you follow the rules of the yoga system, you are doing so with an effort to achieve bliss. This bliss is associated with a divine power that is greater than any earthly being. When you experience enlightenment, you experience life without perception, suffering, and chaos. You eliminate the constant turmoil of your mind and see the true beauty of things. Yoga masters believe that enlightenment takes many lifetimes to achieve, and some believe you experience it through death. For the purpose of childbirth, enlightenment comes from meeting your child for the first time. It is the discipline of using the Yoga Birth Method and following the eight-step pathway. Enlightenment will be how you describe your labor experience.

The Yoga Birth Method Pathway

Now that you have an understanding of the yoga system, let me explain how it will relate to your labor and how it can encourage you have a natural childbirth experience. The practice of yoga leads a person into deeper self-awareness; it provides a sense of social responsibility and acknowledges that divine power exists whether a person discovers it within or as a higher source. When you use the eight steps in labor, this divine connection can be made during your birthing experience.

Here is a preview of how the birth method works. In chapter 5 we will go over each step in full detail.

1. Intent to refrain from negative behavior.

2. Intent to practice positive behavior.

3. Awareness of the body.

4. Using breath to link intent to body.

5. Surrender to the natural process.

6. Mindful connection to each contraction.

7. Embracing a calm state throughout labor.

8. Enlightened experience of relationship between self, child, and divine energy.

First, an intention must be set for your labor experience. You must put some thought into how you want labor to occur and how you plan to manage pain so that you have the best chance at a natural experience. You have a responsibility for your actions and thoughts throughout your labor. Being prepared with your birth intention is a good start to ensuring your birth plan is executed.

Pain is inevitable in labor, but how you perceive and manage that pain is a choice that you can make. Your attitude toward your experience will determine how you labor. Through this method, I am preparing you with a step-by-step guide and encouraging you to manage the work with yoga tools. By understanding how to breathe and how to move the body through contractions in each stage of labor, you give yourself the power to be in control.

When you know that you have emotionally prepared yourself for the experience, then you allow yourself to surrender and let nature take its course. You let go of the attachment to pain and embrace the experience of birth. By acknowledging the experience of pain as necessary for your child to arrive, as we describe the baby's movements in chapter 4, you are better able to directly connect with your child. This gives you the ability to practice concentration and embrace meditation throughout your labor.

In addition, understanding the process of what happens during labor (covered in chapter 6) and what medical interventions may occur (see chapter 7) can help you make informed choices, allowing you to have mindful control over your birth experience. Enlightenment comes as your reward by trusting yourself during this entire process and working with your child as a team.

In order to understand how to use each step, I will explain what happens in the first stage of labor. By being able to identify what is happening in each phase of the first stage physically and mentally, you will know when to apply the appropriate techniques for that phase of progression. We will also cover medical assistance and birth interventions in order to give you the ability to make informed choices during your birth experience. I have included wonderful birth stories from women with very different birth outcomes, and I hope they inspire you to use the Yoga Birth Method and have a beautiful birth journey.

2

Yoga During Pregnancy

There are numerous benefits to practicing yoga during your pregnancy. If you have never taken a class before, you will want to listen to your body physically and practice these postures with ease. When you feel uncomfortable, come out of the pose and take a break. Take time getting in and out of postures, and be mindful of how your baby feels during your practice. There is no rush with yoga. Practicing should feel good and eliminate stress and tension.

When you are pregnant, your body changes. Things you may have been able to do freely before may seem more challenging over the nine months. A rise in pregnancy hormones such as estrogen, progesterone, prolactin, relaxin, and oxytocin also change your body. Yoga can balance hormonal changes and help your body adapt easier to these changes. As your body grows to make room for the baby, postures can help you feel stronger and less heavy. Deep breathing relieves anxiety, stress, and tension, and it prepares you for breathing in labor.

There are different ways that you can add yoga to your daily life during your nine months. You can choose to incorporate specific postures in each trimester or follow a safe routine for the entire duration. I suggest that in addition to practicing any of the postures in this chapter, you also practice the early stage flow two to three times a week. You will learn this posture flow in chapter 6. By incorporating the early stage flow into a daily routine, you will be better prepared to use the sequence in labor.

Over the next nine months you will notice certain changes in your body. I have explained some of these changes for each trimester and included some postures that can help make you feel better. These postures encourage your body to make space for your baby; relieve heartburn; stretch and strengthen achy muscles in the back, shoulders, and legs; relieve cramping of the uterus as it expands; reduce fatigue; and assist with hormones that open muscles and joints required for delivery. Most importantly, yoga increases blood and oxygen flow to the umbilical cord, which nourishes your baby and promotes a healthy start to development. I have outlined the benefits, cautions, and modifications in each pose to help make your practice easier if you are inexperienced. If you have experience with yoga or follow a regular practice, you may find that your pregnant body has some limitations, take your time, listen to your body, feel your baby's reactions, there is no need to push or rush your poses.

Breathing is an important part of a yoga practice. By moving the breath deeply, you can control how you do postures, prevent injury, and identify places in the body that are uncomfortable. In a prenatal yoga practice, we use *Ujjayi*, or ocean, breathing. This breathing technique is done in and out, through the nose, where you create a deep, smooth wave sound at the back of your throat; we like to call it the Darth Vader breath. Close your eyes and imagine you are sitting comfortably in a relaxing place. As you breathe, feel as though you are taking in all the air and the energy around you. Feel your breath moving deep down to your toes. As you exhale, your breath comes all the way back up and releases from your nose. All your tension exhales away with it. This long, deep breath is a way for you take in the relaxing atmosphere and be present. When you practice these postures, use a deep abdominal inhalation and exhalation. By being mindful of your breathing now, you will be able to identify with YBM breathing techniques in labor.

As you practice these postures, you can add Kegel exercises, which help keep the pelvic floor strong. This will help in later months of pregnancy and with the pushing stage of childbirth. By continuous practice of Kegel exercises, you also help with the uterus's postnatal recovery and help prevent postnatal incontinence. There is no required amount of Kegels that can be prescribed. My best advice is to make a habit of doing these simple exercises as many times as you can throughout the day. Some women like to add them to certain things they do daily such as brushing their teeth, showering, cooking, or driving; this way, it becomes part of the daily routine.

To do a Kegel, imagine that you are urinating and midway through it the phone rings, and you have to stop and run to answer the phone. The muscle contraction to stop urinating is the Kegel squeeze. It's important to find the right muscles to tighten. To ensure you have the right muscles, next time you have to urinate, start to go and then stop. Feel the muscles in your vagina, bladder, or anus get tight and lift upward. These are the pelvic floor muscles. If you feel them tighten, you've done the exercise right.

Another component to a yoga practice is mind control or meditation. During your pregnancy, you might be overwhelmed with thoughts and worries along the way. In order to change your thoughts from negative to positive, you can use mantras. These are motivational statements to help you focus on positive outcomes or emotions. By focusing on a weekly mantra, you can replace negative thoughts with feel-good energy thoughts and bring inspirational vibrations into your pregnancy. Mantras are simple words or sentences that you can repeat over and over again. I have included forty mantras in this chapter, one for each week of your pregnancy. If one of them works well for you, then you can use it as much as you like. These man- tras can be used in labor as points of focus in your breathing and to encourage concentration and deep meditation. They work well with birth intentions and create harmony between mind and body.

Your yoga birth experience can start as early as week one of your pregnancy or as soon as you decide to start using the practices in this book. The following poses are easy and safe to use during all three trimesters. By focusing on these postures, you maximize the benefits they offer to that specific trimester. Practice ocean breathing (*Ujjayi*) in each pose and focus on a new mantra each week. You can take your practice off the mat and into your daily life by being aware of your breathing from time to time and repeating your mantra as often as you like to help stimulate good yogic energy.

Before you attempt to practice, make sure you consult your doctor. You will want to make sure that the baby is in good health and that you are aware of any blood-pressure issues, blood-sugar concerns, or physical restrictions.

The First Trimester
weeks 0–14

Your Body
- You have an increased level of estrogen and progesterone in your body, causing nausea and fatigue.

- You have increased blood levels flowing in your body.

- Your uterus feels crampy as it begins to grow.

- Some common complaints may be acne, bleeding gums, bloating, heartburn, headaches, insomnia, and frequent urination.

Your Baby
- The heart forms by week 3.

- The face, eyes, and nose are visible by week 10.

- Fingers and toes are starting to form.

- The brain has begun to form.

- Blood and oxygen begin to flow through the umbilical cord to organs by week 14.

- Hair follicles are growing.

- Your baby weighs 1¾ ounces and is nine centimeters long by week 14.

Mantras for the First Trimester

week

1	I am a goddess of energy carrying a beautiful soul.
2	I am strong and I feel good.
3	I am divine energy surrounded with love.
4	I feel empowered with love.
5	My child is filled with love.
6	My child is growing into a healthy being.
7	My child is divine light.
8	I have no fear of the future as I embrace the present.
9	My body is a gift of light and purity.
10	I am healthy and I feel wonderful.
11	I am surrounded by positive energy.
12	My child is healthy and strong.
13	I am beautiful.
14	I enjoy being pregnant.

It may seem hard to practice in the first trimester if you are feeling tired and uncomfortable. This is a good time to do poses that help you relax and regain some energy. Once you get into a groove of doing a few poses a day, it will encourage you to move and feel good about the months ahead.

In addition to yoga, there are other ways of getting physical activity into your daily routine that will be beneficial to your health and well-being over the duration of your pregnancy. You can try walking twenty minutes two to four times a week, swimming once a week, or mild weight training to help keep your muscles toned. These additional physical exercises will help keep you from feeling fatigued as your body becomes heavier with the weight of the baby. When you lack physical exercise in pregnancy, it is harder to manage the third trimester, when your body carries the most weight. Practicing the postures below and maintaining cardiovascular health will help release positive endorphins and keep you feeling great throughout the entire nine months.

Prenatal Postures for the First Trimester

Balancing Table Pose

How it helps: This pose will increase strength and encourage you to maintain balance in your pregnancy. It will also combat fatigue by increasing oxygen in the brain, which will help the body balance hormone production.

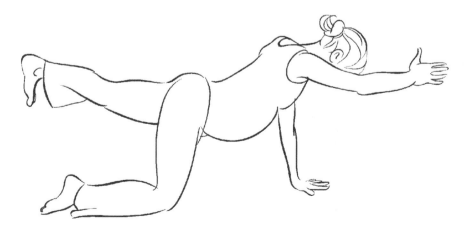

Modifications: If you have wrist pain or carpal tunnel syndrome, make a fist with your hands and avoid applying pressure to your wrists. If you have lower backaches, then extend your leg but keep your toes on the ground.

How to do this pose:

- On your hands and knees in a table position, inhale and lift your right leg up so that it is parallel to the floor. Point your toes backward and exhale.

- Keeping your neck in line with your spine, slowly inhale and bring the left arm up and parallel to the floor. Reach your fingers forward and exhale.

- Using *Ujayyi* breathing, hold the pose for three to six breaths. How long you hold the pose depends on your comfort level. Feel free to hold as little or as long as you wish, but be sure to maintain the same time frame on the opposite side for balance.

- To release, slowly exhale and come back into a table position. Repeat on the opposite arm and leg. Repeat three times on each side and hold for three deep breaths.

Extended Puppy Pose

How it helps: This pose will relieve nausea by allowing you to rest your head. Often nausea and morning sickness occur in pregnancy due to the increased level of hormones in the body such as HCG (human chorionic gonadotropin) and estrogen. Often just eating something light such as salted crackers can help relieve nausea. In addition, Extended Puppy Pose decreases external stimulation and gives you an opportunity to relax and stretch comfortably. It stretches the hips and relieves uterine cramping.

Modifications: If you have headaches or sinus discomfort, make fists and place them under your forehead. If you have any issues with your shoulders, bend your elbows outward and release the extension in your arms.

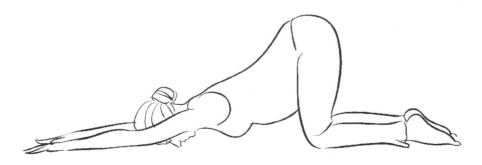

How to do this pose:

- Get on your hands and knees. Keep your shoulders right above your wrists and your hips directly over your knees. Reach your hands forward into a full arm extension and curl your toes beneath you.

- With a deep exhalation, move your butt halfway back, almost to your heels. Your arms should remain active—your elbows should never touch the mat.

- Next, drop your forehead to your mat or to a pillow. Keep your neck relaxed and retain a little curve in your lower back. Press your hands down and then stretch through your arms while pulling your hips back to your heels. Continue breathing into your back and feel your spine lengthening from the neck to the tailbone.

- You can hold the pose for thirty to sixty seconds or even longer if you are comfortable. There is no harm in going up to a minute or more. To exit, release your butt down to your heels.

Happy Baby Pose

How it helps: This pose will relieve nausea by allowing
you to rest your head. It decreases external
stimulation and gives you an opportunity to relax
and stretch comfortably. It stretches the hips and
relieves uterine cramping.

Modifications: If you have difficulty reaching for your
feet, then use a strap or a belt around each foot
instead. If you have any discomfort in your back,
then release one foot to the mat and work one side
at a time.

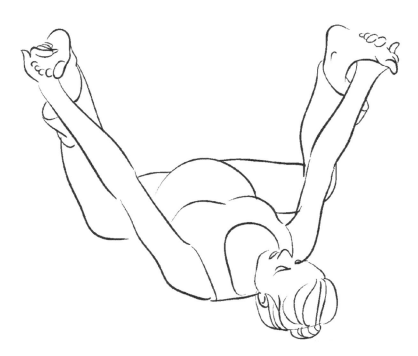

How to do this pose:

- Lie on your back and hold your feet. If you have difficulty holding the feet, hold behind your thighs. Open your knees as you pull your knees toward your armpits.

- Feel the length of your entire spine making contact with the ground.

- Gently press your heels upward as you continue to hold on to your feet.

- Feel your tailbone, spine, and the base of your skull lengthening as you gently stretch.

- Hold the pose for a minute or as long as is comfortable. To release, exhale and slowly move the feet back to the floor.

Gate Pose

How it helps: This pose stretches the side body,
relieving any aches and pains from the uterus
growing. It opens the chest and enables more
oxygen to come into the body. It combats fatigue
and provides energy.

Modifications: If you have issues with your knees, place
a blanket under your knee for support. If you have
sciatica, do not reach all the way over. Keep the arm
extended straight up. Flex the extended toe upward
if you have tension in the knee.

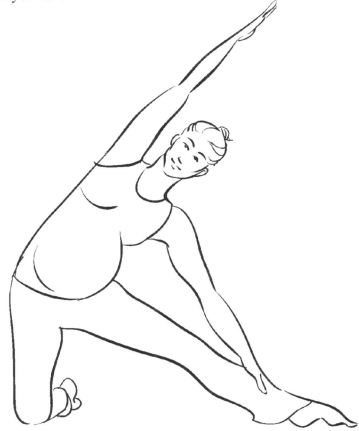

How to do this pose:

- Kneel on the floor. Stretch your right leg out to the right and press the foot to the floor. Turn your upper torso so it's facing forward.

- Bend your left arm up and over your head as you lean toward the right leg. Contract the right side of the torso and stretch the left. Place your right hand on the outer right hip or as far down as comfortable without twisting the shoulder; keep your body aligned as if it were against a wall. Use deep *Ujayyi* breathing as you allow yourself to go deeper on the exhalation.

- Stay in this pose anywhere from thirty seconds to a minute. Come up as you inhale, reaching through the top arm to draw the torso upright. Bring the right knee back beside the left, and repeat with the other leg.

Reclined Hand to Big Toe Pose

How it helps: This pose stretches the inner thighs and opens the hips. Being on your back is easier in the first trimester. Practicing back positions now encourages you to maintain the practice throughout pregnancy, making hip openers easier as your body gets bigger and your baby grows.

Modifications: If you have difficulty reaching for your foot, hold behind your thigh. If you have issues with your shoulders, use a belt or strap around your foot.

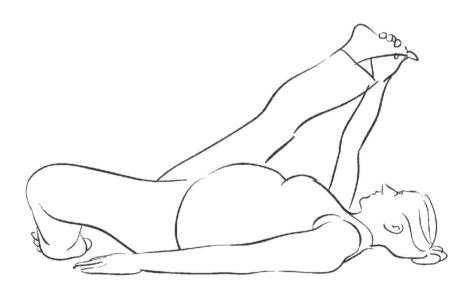

How to do this pose:

- As you lie on your back, raise the right leg and bend the left knee to the side.

- Take hold of either the right big toe with the right hand or use a strap around the foot and hold the lower ends of the strap with the right hand. If needed, place the left hand on the left thigh to encourage the hips to stay down.

- Extend the right leg out to the side. Keep the hips on the floor and use deep *Ujayyi* breathing.

- Hold this position for several breaths. Repeat the pose on the other side, taking care to hold it for the same length of time.

Reclined Lord of the Dance Pose

How it helps: This pose stretches the hip flexor and
   opens the chest. It opens the lungs and allows
   oxygen and blood to better flow throughout the
   entire body. It reduces nausea and heartburn by
   opening the diaphragm and creating space in the
   esophagus.

Modifications: If you have any wrist pains or carpal
   tunnel syndrome, use a strap around your foot. If
   you have a lower backache, avoid pulling the foot
   back toward you.

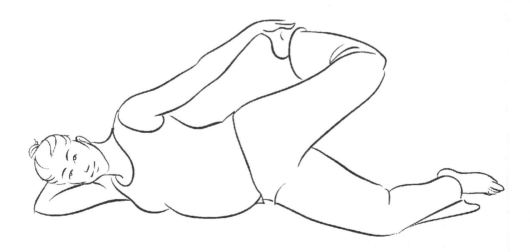

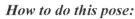

How to do this pose:

- Lie on your side with your left arm comfortably under your head.

- Bend the knees and grab your right ankle behind you with your right hand.

- Press your foot into your hand to stretch the front of the leg and the shoulder. Use *Ujayyi* breathing and press the foot into the hand on the exhalation.

- Hold for three to four breaths and release; repeat on the other side.

The Second Trimester
weeks 15–27

Your Body
- Breasts are starting to produce colostrum.
- You may have gained approximately 5 to 10 pounds.
- You can feel your baby move after 24 weeks.
- You may start to feel back pain.
- You may start to feel sciatic nerve pain. The sciatic nerve is a major nerve connecting from the mid back slightly above the hip and all the way down to the sole of the foot. Pressure on this nerve can cause severe pain throughout the entire leg.

Your Baby
- Eyelids can open and close.
- All the nerves have developed.
- Can hear sounds at week 18.
- Has taste buds at week 22.
- Sex organs begin to develop and are visible at week 20.
- Tooth buds begin to form.
- Will respond to pokes at the abdomen.

Mantras for the Second Trimester

week

15	I am glowing with love.
16	I am empowered with strength.
17	My body is a temple of love.
18	My child is beautiful.
19	My body is beautiful.
20	I am aware of this moment.
21	I love my life.
22	All things are as they should be.
23	My baby is happy.
24	I can do anything.
25	I embrace each moment with joy.
26	I feel blessed.
27	I feel fantastic.

The second trimester is your "personal power" trimester. In the coming weeks you will be stronger and feel beautiful as you carry your child. Do poses that bring out your inner strength and vitalize you. Take advantage of feeling great, and maximize your ability to practice. In addition to working through these poses, in chapter 6 you will learn the early stage flow. Once you are comfortable with the early stage flow, the sequence can be added to your routine.

Prenatal Postures for the Second Trimester

Tree Pose

How it helps: This pose will help you continue
to maintain balance and strength during your
pregnancy. It opens the hips and chest, encouraging
a deep connection to breath and vitality.

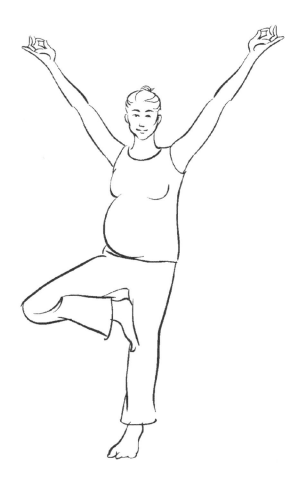

Modifications: If you have any balancing issues, use a wall or support yourself with a chair. For beginners, keep your foot at your ankle and do not raise it until you are comfortable.

How to do this pose:

- In a standing position, shift your weight to the right side.

- Lift the sole of your left foot to the inside of your right leg. Place it on your ankle, shin, or inner thigh. Avoid placing your foot on your knee.

- Lift your hands up and square your hips forward.

- Press the sole of your foot into your leg to create resistance. You can use deep breathing here and hold for as long as comfortable. You can use a wall for support.

- Release and switch sides.

Chair Pose

How it helps: This pose will help you continue
to maintain balance and strength during your
pregnancy. It strengthens the lower back and core
to prevent aches and pains. Use deep breathing and
connect to your sense of inner power.

Modifications: If you have discomfort in the knees,
support your back against a wall and lower yourself
slowly. If you have any injuries in your shoulders, do
not raise your arms above your head.

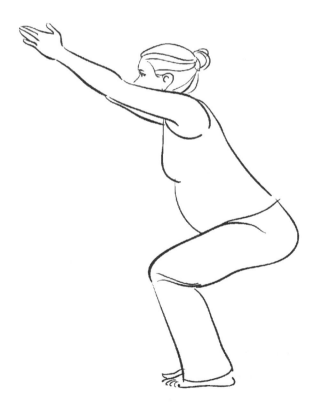

How to do this pose:

- Stand with your feet hip-distance apart.

- Come into a semi-squat and raise your arms.

- Keep your back straight and your core strong.

- Look forward and relax your shoulders. Use deep breathing and sink lower as you exhale. On the inhale you can lift up slightly and lower again on the next exhalation.

- Release to a standing forward bend and repeat.

Lord of the Dance Pose

How it helps: This pose will help you continue to maintain balance and strength during your pregnancy. It opens the hips and chest, encouraging a deep connection to breath and vitality. It safely strengthens the abdominals to help prepare for postnatal recovery.

Modifications: If you have any wrist pain or carpal tunnel syndrome, use a strap or belt around your ankle. Support yourself with a wall or chair if necessary. Bend your standing leg if you have any knee problems.

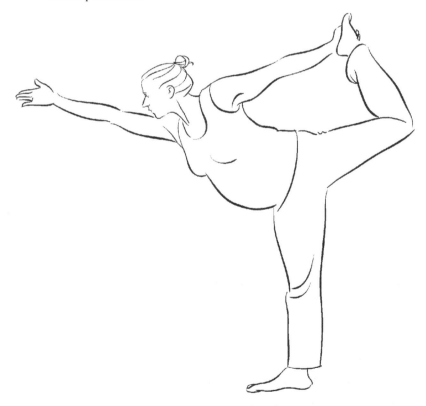

How to do this pose:

- Stand upright with your weight balanced between both legs, then shift your weight to your right leg.

- Raise your left foot behind you, and reach back and grab your foot with your left hand.

- Press your foot behind you and extend.

- Open your shoulders and keep your hips square.

- Reach your right hand forward. Hold for four breaths.

- Release and switch sides.

Seated Wide-Angle Forward Bend Pose

How it helps: This pose will help stretch inner thighs and hips. It lengthens the spine and releases back tension.

Modifications: For any back issues, be sure to bend forward slowly. Do not go too deep if you feel tension in the groin or hips. Place pillows under the hips if your lower back feels tight.

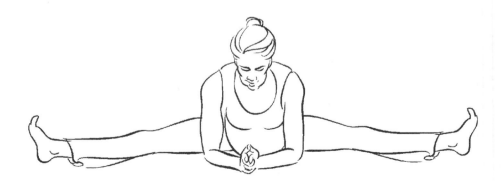

How to do this pose:

- Sit comfortably and extend your legs outward.

- Flex your toes and press your heels out.

- Bend forward and keep your spine straight. Extend from the chest. Use *Ujayyi* breathing and ease into the stretch on the exhalation.

- Your hands and elbows should align with your shoulders; this helps to keep the spine straight. Hold for thirty seconds.

Side Plank Pose

How it helps: This pose will help strengthen the upper body and core. It helps to prevent aches and pains. It will help you connect to a sense of inner power.

Modifications: If you have any wrist pain or carpal tunnel syndrome, make a fist with your hands and avoid applying pressure to your wrists. If you have lower backaches, then bring your extended leg slightly forward.

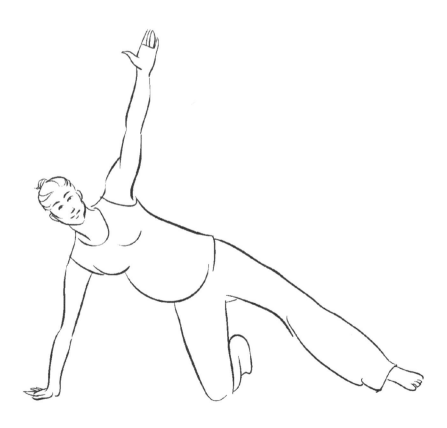

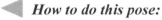 ***How to do this pose:***

- From Table Pose, turn outward to balance on your right knee and right hand.

- Extend your left leg out.

- Keep your hips rotating upward and extend your left hand upward. Use *Ujayyi* breathing and maintain your balance.

- Hold for thirty seconds and switch sides.

Camel Pose

How it helps: This pose will help relieve diaphragm pressure. It stretches the shoulders from carrying baby weight forward and opens the hips. It encourages oxygen intake and strengthens the abdominals to help prepare for postnatal recovery.

Modifications: For lower back pain or injuries, do not bend back deeply. Keep your back straight and just release the head. For knee discomfort, keep a blanket or pillow under the knees.

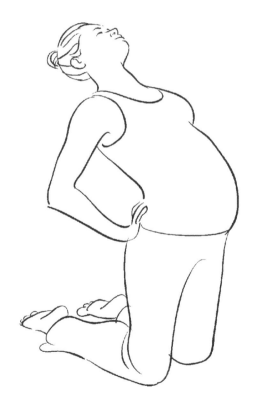

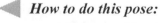 ***How to do this pose:***

- Align your hips with your knees.

- Place your hands on your lower back.

- Press your elbows toward each other and let your
  head relax backward. Use deep *Ujjayi* breathing
  and press the hips forward on the exhalation.

- Keep pushing your hips forward
  and hold for four breaths.

The Third Trimester
weeks 28–40

Your Body

- You may feel lower backaches.

- You may feel pressure in the pelvis as your baby drops after 32 weeks.

- Your diaphragm will feel squeezed, and it may seem harder to breathe deeply.

- You may start to experience Braxton Hicks contractions.

- Your ankles may feel swollen.

- It may seem harder to move around.

- Hormones begin to develop to produce breast milk.

Your Baby

- Can focus and blink.

- Lanugo—the fine, hairlike particles that protect your baby from the amniotic fluid—begins to shed at week 39.

- Lungs fully develop at week 37.

- Your baby may weigh from 6 to 9 pounds and be 14 to 15 inches long.

Mantras for the Third Trimester

week

28   I am calm and peaceful.

29   I trust my body.

30   My body feels strong.

31   I am patient and calm.

32   I love my body.

33   I am surrounded with support.

34   I am in control of my thoughts.

35   I am ready to be a mother.

36   I enjoy each breath.

37   I feel wonderful.

38   My baby is healthy and ready to be born.

39   My body is strong and ready for labor.

40   My baby and I are a team.

In the remaining weeks of the final trimester, you should be getting ready to give birth. You can use any of the postures from the first and second trimester. Make sure that you are practicing the early stage flow as much as you can. How you carry yourself can have an effect on your baby's positioning. You want to encourage your baby to move into head-down vertex position around week thirty-four. Your care provider will begin to monitor positioning in the last few weeks of pregnancy. It's important to not spend too much time in reclined positions or lying on your back for prolonged periods of time to avoid breech or occiput posterior position.

In the third trimester, spend more time practicing deeper hip openers and focusing on pelvic muscles. Being able to maintain fluidity and movement will help you manage posture transitioning in labor through contractions. If you have maintained a regular practice throughout your pregnancy, you should feel mobile and flexible in your last trimester. Feeling strong and relaxed in the last few weeks will definitely give you a head start in using the YBM *asanas* during labor. However, starting these poses at any point in pregnancy will always be beneficial. As the saying goes, better late than never!

Prenatal Postures for the Third Trimester

In the third trimester you can use all of the previous poses. I strongly encourage you to practice the early stage flow in the final trimester to make sure you are maintaining your mobility (see chapter 6). By practicing regularly, it will be easier to come into the flow during labor. You and your partner can use the hands-on techniques in the partner support chapter (chapter 8) to help make these poses more comfortable in the last months of pregnancy.

The Side-Lying Pose (below) is a reminder for you to rest on your side and not on your back. Rest one hand on the lower back and massage, and use the other hand on the neck to release tension.

Side-Lying Pose

How it helps: This pose will encourage anterior positioning. This position is when the baby's head is down and the baby is facing mom's spine. It is the optimal birth position because it facilitates an easier delivery.

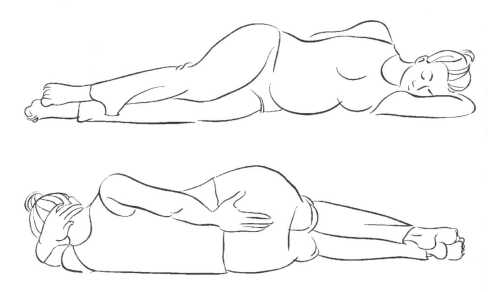

3

Demystifying the Fear of Childbirth

When a woman discovers she is pregnant, she becomes excited, especially if it was a planned pregnancy. Soon after the excitement, though, fear and worry may set in—about the health of the baby, weight gain, financial resources, relationship changes, how the labor will go, the pain she can't identify with, and the fear about possible delivery problems. This list can go on and on, and every woman worries about different things. The idea behind this book is to help you understand what happens in labor and empower you with yoga tools to make it as natural as possible and to make informed decisions during the entire process. My goal is to eliminate worry and shift your thoughts to a trusted birth experience.

Labor pain cannot be described in black-and-white detail. Pain is relative to each person who feels it. The key to pain management is to understand your pain tolerance and threshold. Knowing how you react to pain will help you build pain tolerance in labor. Knowing that there is a progression in labor will help you pass thresholds. When labor begins, the pain may seem intolerable, but the first phase of contractions is only the beginning. I like to think of early labor as a teaser. If you prepare yourself for the levels of pain, then getting through the stages naturally is achievable. How do you begin to understand the levels of pain and at the same time eliminate some of the stress and worry? Educate yourself about birth—how you can bring concentration into your experience and how meditation can help you remain calm and in control—and recognize when to practice sense withdrawal. When you understand how to use the YBM tools for pain management, you will have a better chance at achieving a natural birth.

Let's look at some of the questions you may have during your pregnancy that generally tend to initiate fear.

What is normal birth?

Normal birth happens when a woman starts contractions between her thirty-seventh and forty-second week of pregnancy. The pregnancy is considered low risk and without complications. "Low risk" means that the mother is healthy and under the age of thirty-five. The baby is in the vertex (head down), anterior position. There would be no reason for medical interference. Normal birth does not necessarily mean natural birth.

What is natural birth?

Natural birth means that the woman has no medication or medical intervention during her birthing process. Her contractions start on their own, effacement and dilation progress without medical assistance, and she is able to manage the pain effectively. Natural birth eliminates drugs' side effects such as nausea, lack of movement, fetal or maternal distress, and fetal grogginess after delivery.

What is a complicated labor?

A complicated labor may happen for many reasons. Complications are called dystocias and could cause a woman's labor to require medical interference.

Here are situations that would be considered complications:

1. Arrest of active labor—When the cervix dilates to four or five centimeters, the progression of dilation should speed up at this point. However, sometimes it does not and may take longer than usual. If dilation slows in active labor, it is called protracted labor. If it stops for more than two hours, it is called arrested labor. If a woman does not resume contractions, then induction or cesarean section might be necessary.

2. Uterine inertia—This occurs when there is a problem with contraction timing and strength. The contractions are not strong or long enough to dilate the cervix.

3. Cephalo-pelvic disorder—The baby's head is bigger than the mother's pelvis, and the baby may not be able to descend through the pelvic structure.

4. Complications with the fetus—The baby may experience complications prior to the start of labor. Sometimes these complications present themselves during labor. Such complications could be a prolapsed cord (when the umbilical cord descends into the cervix before the baby; this can be fatal if the baby puts pressure on the cord and cuts off blood and oxygen supply), breech position, or fetal distress that can cause macomium secretions. Macomium is the first stool that baby will eliminate after birth; it is the collection of particles the baby swallows during time in utero. Sometimes the baby will eliminate this waste into the amniotic fluid during labor and possibly swallow it. The ingestion of macomium can lead to emergency respiratory issues.

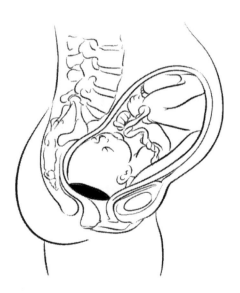

5. Maternal distress—The mother is suffering from anxiety, fear, and exhaustion, which causes her body to react by contracting muscles and slowing the process of dilation and effacement.

How long will labor last?

It would be wonderful if this was a standard textbook answer. The truth is that labor is different for every woman; in fact, no woman will experience the same labor twice. Labor is like DNA: everyone's is different. There are some textbook facts that can help you understand the length of time a woman may need to birth her child or the reason labor can be long. Here is a general list:

1. First baby—If this is your first baby, then your body has to learn how to give birth. The entire process is new. The cervix will be dilating and effacing for the first time and may need the extra time to figure it out. Often second babies (and thereafter) do not take as long, because the body has been trained and knows how to get through the process.

2. Cervical conditions—If your cervix is thick and firm, then it will take longer to get 100 percent effaced and ten centimeters dilated, as opposed to a woman who starts with a thin and soft cervix prior to labor beginning.

3. Cephalo-pelvic proportion—If your baby is too large for the dimensions of your pelvis, it could cause a slow-starting labor or, as mentioned earlier, cause problems in the active phase of labor.

4. Baby's positioning—Your baby needs to be in a head-down position facing your spine. This is called occipital anterior and considered natural birth position.

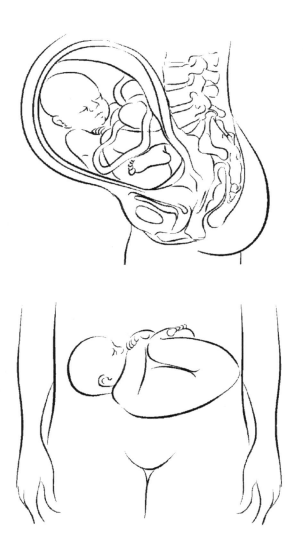

However, this does not mean that labor time will be quick. It only eliminates the need for intervention.

If the baby is breech (head up, butt down) or occipital posterior or transverse, it may cause labor time to be longer and more painful due to the difficulty in having the baby move through the birth canal. Sometimes a woman may experience back labor (back discomfort or pain during labor) when the baby is entering the birth canal in an unnatural position. Back labor can be felt when the baby is creating pressure on the hip joints or muscles in the lower back region.

5. Mother distress—If you are stressed or exhausted in labor, then you will play a part in the timing of your labor. When you show signs of stress, you cause the muscles to tighten. This will restrict oxygen and blood flow to the baby. Lack of oxygen slows the dilation process. Stress causes the body to function in fight-or-flight mode, kicking in the sympathetic nervous system. It's important to maintain a calm state in labor, using relaxation and breathing exercises to keep the body in the parasympathetic mode, or resting state. This is the reason comfort measures and different laboring techniques are used. The Yoga Birth Method guides you to be in the relaxed state throughout the entire course of labor.

Breech position, top
Occipital posterior or transverse, bottom

How will I know I am in labor?

This is the question that pregnant women ask for nine months. They ask their moms, doctors, and friends who have been through it. The truth is everyone starts labor differently. The only way to know for sure is when you experience contractions that don't go away—and, of course, the end result will be a baby in your arms!

But there are many different signs that will signal either possible labor or true labor. The key is to know the difference. By educating yourself to be ready, you reduce anxiety, worry, and fear. You take yourself out of the darkness and spend your time waiting for labor in the light. The last month of pregnancy is an anxious one for sure, especially if you experience Braxton Hicks contractions off and on. The best way to get through the anticipation is to spend your time getting your body relaxed. Let go of the fear and accept that regardless of how much you worry, you can't prevent labor from happening.

There are many books on the laboring process. There are also many classes you can take that teach childbirth education. Your birthing hospital will also have these classes available for you. There are some sure, tell-tale signs that labor has started. However, it is a waiting and guessing game. One piece of advice is not to get caught up in the preliminary phase of labor. If you are feeling contractions and they are far apart and seem infrequent, then get busy. Start the yoga flow for early stage labor that you will learn in chapter 6, go to the movies, clean the house, and go out for dinner—or sleep! Pretend you are not in labor. If you expect baby to arrive soon after early labor begins, then this will definitely extend your actual laboring time and emotionally exhaust you.

What if I can't do it naturally and need an epidural?

Don't worry about this. Put this thought out of your head. When you set out to experience a natural birth, you have no idea what to expect. No one can explain to you how the contractions will feel. There are a few tricks that can help you build pain tolerance. Try holding a piece of ice in your hand for sixty seconds, then take a break for two minutes and do it again, holding for ninety seconds. This technique gives you some idea of managing pain. However, the feeling of the ice is not even close to labor pain!

The fact that you want to do your best to experience natural labor is a good start. Being prepared and equipped with the coping tools in the birth method is your step in the right direction. If it happens that you must take medications in your labor, this does not make you a failure. It doesn't change your experience for the worst. Learning to accept the process as it unfolds in the moment is important. Practicing surrender is your way of accepting that sometimes things don't work out as planned. We will discuss the waterfall effect and emotions later.

4

Managing the Big Day

Labor happens in three stages: first stage, pushing stage, and placenta delivery. The first stage consists of three phases: early, active, and transition. The Yoga Birth Method is designed to take you through the first and second stage until the baby is born. When you use the techniques through the early, active, and transition phases, it will help you manage the increasing intensity of contractions and also encourage progression toward the second stage effectively.

Each phase in the first stage has emotional and physical signs that are similar for everyone. Even though your labor will be completely different from someone else's, there are similar signs that can help identify where a laboring woman may be in the process to reach ten-centimeter dilation and 100 percent effacement. This means the cervix has opened to a full ten-centimeter diameter and has thinned out completely to 100 percent.

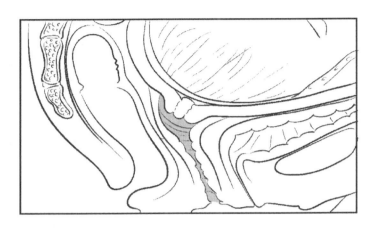

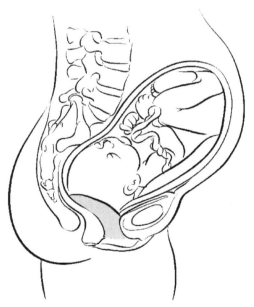

The contractions that occur during labor are muscles in the abdomen pushing baby in a downward motion to enable the cervix to open. As contractions get stronger and more frequent, they bring baby closer to delivery. Now, this does not imply that strong contractions two minutes apart mean baby will be born in an hour. It means that labor is definitely progressing naturally and that the contractions are effective enough for vaginal delivery. As you know, labor is different for every woman. There is no way to categorize labor and predict how long it will take. We can only look at the generalization of physical and emotional changes that happen in each stage of labor. In order to understand what happens in labor, it's important for you to understand that your baby is working as hard as the pain you are feeling. Your baby needs the intensity and frequency of contractions because it must make six cardinal movements to complete birth. As you progress through the first stage, your baby is reaching milestones in the descent toward the birth canal. As your baby progresses through these movements, the contractions change and intensify to help them get through tighter spots in your pelvis. The reason some women decide to use pain medication is to avoid the pain they feel, they are so engaged in the pain and how it is affecting them, without associating the pain to the process of baby's descent toward the world. The baby cannot avoid pain, in fact when medication slows and weakens the contractions the baby will not be able to decent to birth. When you realize that pain equals baby's progress, it makes it easier to choose a natural path to delivery.

◀ *Closed cervix, top*
Fully dilated cervix, bottom

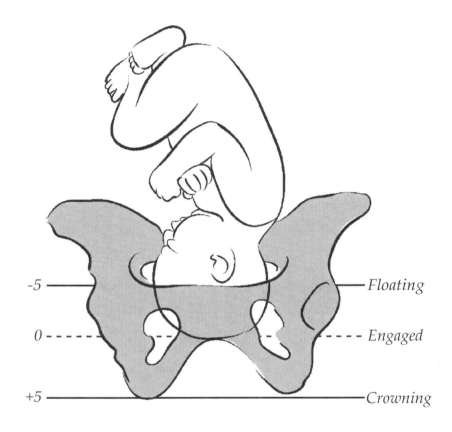

-5 —————— *Floating*

0 - - - - - - - - - - - - *Engaged*

+5 —————— *Crowning*

Your baby makes six cardinal movements during the first stage of labor:

- descent
- flexion
- internal rotation
- extension
- external rotation
- expulsion

Your cervix responds with three important changes to make room for these movements:

- effacement
- dilation
- anterior tilting

When the baby and cervix are responding in harmony, it is called natural progression. Let's look at this in detail.

You may feel light contractions starting in the weeks prior to labor. These types of contractions are called Braxton Hicks contractions and are considered false labor. These contractions are necessary to help to begin softening and ripening your cervix walls, preparing it for effacement. When true labor begins, regular contractions will start the effacement and dilation process. Each contraction will help the cervix open or dilate toward a ten-centimeter diameter and the cervix walls to thin out. The cervix walls must go from a thick state to a paper-thin state and is measured from 0 to 100 percent completion. Your cervix must also tilt forward, which means it must move from a posterior to an anterior position.

As the cervix makes these changes, your baby works harmoniously by going through the cardinal movements. The movements are measured against the position of the pelvis (see opposite page).

Engagement occurs when your baby's head drops in the pelvis. Progression through labor is measured by the Ischial Spine, which are the pointed notches of the pelvis (see illustration on page 76). Knowing pelvic placement of baby can help make better decisions during labor.

The first movement your baby will make during labor is descent. Baby will move down into the birth canal past zero station. This will occur during early to active phase in stage one labor. Your baby will then make their second move, which is flexion. The baby must tuck chin to chest in order squeeze through the smaller part of the pelvis. Once the baby flexes, they can then make their third movement of internal rotation. The baby must make a half-turn from facing your side body to facing your spine. This is called moving from occipital transverse to occipital anterior. Sometimes this takes a while or doesn't happen. When a baby moves posterior (facing your belly), this could cause back labor, which is really intense and painful. A sign of experiencing back labor is when you feel pressure in the lower back area, either on the right or left side. Back labor can be felt even when not experiencing a contraction. Before delivery some nurses and doctors will let you wait and encourage you to move and change positions to help baby make the turn to anterior. At this point you are in active to transition phase of the first stage.

When the baby is ready to be born, they make the last three movements. These movements occur in stage two labor, called the pushing stage. Baby will extend the head and neck through the birth canal. When this happens, it is called crowning at pelvic station +3. The head may be visible as you begin to push. Once you have pushed your baby's head out, the baby will then make another movement, called external rotation. If the anterior rotation is made, your baby should be facing down as the head is birthed. When the baby's head is born, they will rotate to face sideways. The doctor will usually help your baby make this move. At this point the baby is ready to make the last movement, which is full delivery.

You must be wondering how you will know when all of this is happening. It is difficult to know where the baby and cervix are in the labor process unless your cervix is checked by a nurse, midwife, or ob-gyn. Your responsibility is to know when your labor has started. If you are sure you are in labor, then you can assume your baby and cervix are making progression.

There are times when labor does not progress, and this is termed as dystocia or failure to progress. If this occurs during your labor, there may be a need for medical intervention. The Yoga Birth Method gives you the tools you need to help labor advance. However, being educated on your choices when things seem to take a different direction gives you the power to make the right decisions and still be in control of your birth story.

Experiencing the Start of Labor

As Braxton Hicks contractions come and go in your last weeks of pregnancy, you will be on edge waiting for one of those false contractions to feel real. As mentioned earlier, true labor is identified by contractions that are strong, regular, and create change in the cervix. You can't possibly know if your cervix is changing, but you can identify the three phases of the first stage by becoming familiar with the changes that occur physically and emotionally.

Every woman is different when it comes to pain management. You may find early labor painful if you have a weak tolerance to physical discomfort or you may find early labor to be easier than you expected. The physical and emotional signs below are by no means cut-and-dried for everyone. They are textbook signs that most women experience. As a labor doula, I have seen these signs firsthand. Of course, every woman enters labor differently, with different reactions to the onset of those first contractions. Knowing whether you are starting in the early phase or right into active labor will be your best guess with the first baby. By trusting your body and your knowledge of all the information you received, all you can do is have faith in your labor and use the YBM technique that seems suitable to how you are feeling.

When you know how to identify the stages of labor, you will be able to use the techniques in this handbook to encourage a faster progression for your cervix and your baby's birth. Let's look at an outline of the physical and emotional signs you may experience during each phase of labor. We will go into these signs in more detail as we cover the YBM techniques later.

Early Labor Phase

Usually with the first baby, labor is expected to last anywhere from twelve to twenty-four hours. It is not uncommon for labor to go to forty-eight hours or even longer. Some women even experience pre-labor well before they start early labor. Pre-labor occurs when you start to feel contractions regularly and then they stop unexpectedly and return intermittently. Eventually these contractions progress into first stage. Pre-labor does not start any significant dilation, but it does begin to soften up your cervix for actual labor.

These contractions will seem stronger than your Braxton Hicks contractions and will seem like there is a regular pattern. If you don't know how to identify pre-labor, you might assume that labor is beginning and rush to the hospital. Inevitably, you will be sent home! The entire concept behind the Yoga Birth Method is to teach you not to panic but to trust yourself and your body to know what to do. The anticipation in pre-labor can be frustrating, confusing, and even exhausting if it goes on for a long time. With pre-labor, when you get up and walk around, the contractions usually will subside. Movement in labor, by contrast, creates stronger contractions, and it is the ultimate test to comparing false labor with true labor.

The YBM techniques will give you the knowledge you need to get your contractions from pre-labor to active labor as quickly and naturally as possible.

Typical Signs of True Labor:
- You may experience a dull pain in the lower back and notice it move to the abdomen.

- When you time these pains, there is a regular pattern.

- Your water may start to leak or break—keep in mind that water does not always break on its own in labor.

- Your pains get stronger with movement.

The following are normal physical signs that let you know your labor could be around the corner. Notice how short the list is. Often these pre-labor signs occur in the days before labor starts:

- You may feel the need to clean or organize your house; this is called a nesting urge.

- You may feel like you have the flu and experience nausea, diarrhea, or vomiting.

- You may feel more tired than usual.

These signs don't always occur for every woman but are considered common pre-labor signs—Mother Nature's way of getting you ready for childbirth.

Steady contractions are one of the physical signs of labor. In order to manage pain intensity during labor progression, it's important that you be educated on levels of pain. In early labor, the pain you will experience is just the beginning. As you move into active and transition stage, the pain will progressively intensify. The contractions become longer, stronger, and closer together. When you start to feel that the pain is becoming intolerable, remind yourself that it will get worse. This will help you to keep pain in perspective. By acknowledging the pain as a process to getting to delivery stage, you empower yourself with acceptance. Expecting the pain to progress helps you build a higher pain threshold.

What happens to my body in early labor?

Physical changes in early labor:

- Your cervix will dilate from 1 to 4 centimeters.

- Your contractions may last anywhere from 30 to 45 seconds.

- Your contractions will get progressively longer and stronger.

- This phase can last anywhere from a few hours to twenty hours or more. This can be the longest part of the dilation process.

- Your baby's head will be engaged as baby descends into your pelvis.

When you assume that you are in early labor, use the early stage flow in chapter 6. This sequence can also be used during pre-labor to help encourage contractions into a true labor pattern.

Emotional signs in early labor:

- When you recognize contractions, you will become excited that delivery time has arrived.

- You may start to feel nervous about the labor.

- If you are not prepared for contraction discomfort, you may start to get anxious and develop tension in your body, which could lead to labor distress.

- You may be talkative and energetic from adrenaline hormones rushing through your body.

Once you have spent some time in early labor and your cervix has reached the four-centimeter milestone, your body will begin to experience intense changes. You will notice the contractions are not the same as the ones you were dealing with the past few hours. At some point the contractions should get stronger and closer together as the baby descends into the pelvis toward the birthing canal. Each contraction is necessary to create the pressure of pushing baby further down. As your baby descends, the cervix will keep opening and thinning.

Active labor is considered good labor. If you decide to go to the hospital and your cervix has dilated over four centimeters, you would be admitted into hospital care. If you are less than four centimeters, the hospital staff will most likely send you home until "good" labor has begun. Knowing this, it is your job to manage your labor from the very beginning at home to ensure that you make the right decision as to when to go to the hospital. Using the YBM in early labor will get you into a yogini groove so that you can stay at home as long as possible. By using the YBM sequence in early labor, you start to work with your contractions and your baby to get into active labor sooner.

Active Labor Phase

What happens to my body in active labor?

Physical changes in active labor:

- Your cervix effaces between 90 and 100 percent.

- Dilation can be from 4 to 8 centimeters.

- Your contractions can be 3 to 7 minutes apart.

- Sometimes contractions can have a bouncing pattern between 2 and 15 minutes apart, with an intensity that is much stronger than early labor.

- Your contractions can last 30 to 60 seconds.

- Your contractions should get more painful, with greater intensity in the peak.

- You may not be able to walk or
  talk during a contraction.

- This phase may last from 30 minutes to 10 hours
  or more. Even though labor is active, it may take
  a while to reach transition with first baby.

Emotional signs of active labor:
- If you experienced pre-labor and then went into early
  labor, you may start to feel exhausted and weak.

- You may start to feel frustrated with the progression
  if you haven't managed the contractions well.

- You may feel uncomfortable with the
  contraction intensity causing you to feel
  sadness or anger toward your labor.

- Without proper tools to manage pain, you may
  begin to lose confidence in natural methods.

- Your pain tolerance may begin to diminish if
  you have been in labor for a long time.

During this stage you may start to lose control of your emotions. If you have had a long early labor phase, frustration and exhaustion may start to set in. Once you allow those emotions to get the best of you, it becomes very difficult to manage your birth. If you succumb to the pain, then you might end up making choices that lead you to an assisted birth. Labor can be a marathon, and the only way to prepare for it is through education and preparation. If you are mindful of your emotions, you can start to use coping strategies to help you find ways to get rest even though you may be experiencing intense pain. Managing natural childbirth is not easy, and active labor can become your first hurdle of frustration.

Let me reiterate that medical assistance does not mean failure. Sometimes a woman needs pain medication to help gather her strength and prevent stress on the baby. In other situations, an epidural is used to help baby make a turn from posterior to anterior in the transition stage or to help baby descend. There are valid reasons for making decisions that involve progression medically. Being in control of your labor is important in making those critical decisions. If you made the choice to use the Yoga Birth Method, you will be more likely to stay focused through your difficult emotions. YBM is a natural birthing choice whose techniques can still be used when medical assistance has been received. Later we will discuss the waterfall effect of choices and how YBM can be effective in some of those choices.

When a woman passes the active stage and enters transition, she is almost there! Transition is the final stage before she begins to push her baby out. The cervix must go through its final change to make room for the baby. Transition can be the most difficult phase of labor, but it is also the shortest. The contractions do not get more painful, but they do get more frequent and intense. Making it through active labor without pain medication is another huge milestone. At this point you may feel like you're between a rock and a hard place, where you can no longer go without pain medication. At this stage, depending on where the cervix is dilated and effaced, it may be too late to receive medication, which is a good thing. If your cervix is at 9 centimeters, why would you give in to medication and reverse all your hard work? The time from eight to ten centimeters doesn't take very long; on average, it could be anywhere from thirty minutes to three hours without an epidural.

Staying in a yoga groove is really important during transition. By maintaining a calm, meditative state, you will have a better chance at controlling your pain tolerance during transition.

Transition Phase

What happens to my body in transition?

Physical changes in transition:

- Your cervix dilates from 8 to 10 centimeters.

- Your contractions will be very intense and close together.

- They could be 1 to 3 minutes apart and last 60 to 90 seconds.

- These contractions peak quickly and may have multiple peaks before the next one.

- If your water has not broken, it may rupture in transition.

- There may be a point in transition where your cervix is fully dilated but not completely effaced. Part of the cervical lining may be remaining. This is called a lip and is quite common at 10 cm. In some circumstances, the nurses may massage this lip away during a contraction or they may have you begin to push while pressing the last part of cervix lining away.

- You will feel rectal pressure, causing a feeling of needing to push (the baby is in the birth canal and the head is pressing down; it is important to *not* push to prevent serious vaginal swelling).

- Your legs may begin to shake uncontrollably from the pressure of the baby on your nerves.

- You may feel hot during a contraction and cold right after.

- You will feel nauseous and may vomit.

Emotional signs of transition:

- You may start to feel like giving up.
- The intensity of pain may make you irritable and not want to be touched.
- You may become forgetful and disorientated.
- You will have difficulty moving or communicating.
- You may have a sense of isolation and feel that no one understands your pain.

Once a woman passes through transition, she is ready to begin the pushing stage. We will cover the pushing stage after we go through the techniques of the Yoga Birth Method for the first stage of labor. Now that you have some idea of what to expect during labor, it's a good time to begin covering the Yoga Birth Method and how it helps you through each phase. We will go over the technique in detail, and I will explain how it specifically addresses each phase in the first stage.

5

How to Have an Enlightened Birth

This part of the book will teach you how to give birth. Believe it or not, there is a right way and a wrong way to give birth. The right way is going through labor educated on the process, and the wrong way is avoiding the topic of labor out of fear for the nine months of your pregnancy. Being educated does not always mean you will have 100 percent control of your birth. It means that you have the knowledge and the resources to make the right decisions for you and your baby. Education gives you the tools you need to choose a birthing method to assist your labor. You have decided to research your options for a natural birth, and that is the reason you are holding this book. Even though you may have your doubts as to whether you can manage the unknown pain, let me assure you natural childbirth is possible. It happens all over the world every day. The Yoga Birth Method will make your birth a positive and natural experience. The technique adapts specifically to the emotional and physical changes in each stage of labor that we covered in the previous chapter. It provides you with a program that enables you to progress through each stage with the knowledge you need to manage the changes that are happening to your body.

Getting on the Path: Setting the Intention

The Yoga Birth Method is an eight-step birthing pathway. This pathway is a complete outline to your childbirth journey. Your pathway begins with setting a birth intention. This birth intention is going to be your direct link to your child and the motivation you will need to manage your birth story the entire way through. Your intention will connect you to your birth experience before it begins because you will be planning your intentions prior to labor starting.

In other birthing methods, women are asked to remove themselves from their pain. They are asked to meditate on something external, such as being on a beach or in a beautiful place. I believe that this type of coping strategy is short-lived during labor. As pain progresses, it is hard to disassociate from it. As contractions become stronger, it will become difficult to tune the physical body out and imagine sitting on a beach. Contractions are painful, and their purpose is to push baby into the birthing canal and help you dilate and efface. When these very important things are happening to your body, you need to be present and awake to them. You need to be mindful of your contractions so that you can be connected to your baby and the movements baby is making. Your child is also on a birth pathway. By meditating on something external and trying to force your mind to be elsewhere, you lose that direct link to your own experience. Besides, imagine sitting on a beach while thunder and lightning are all around you and rain is crashing down on you. It is not fun or relaxing.

Birth intentions in the YBM practice become your meditative focus points. They resonate with you because you choose them based on your personality.

What is an intention?

A working definition for intention is "to have in mind a purpose or plan, to direct the mind, to aim." Lacking intention, we sometimes stray without meaning or direction, but with it, all the forces of the universe can align to make even the most impossible, possible. Your intention for the YBM pathway will set the tone for your birth story. The idea is to experience birth as a mindful and enlightened way to bring your child into the world. To make that possible, you need to have an action plan. You can also use mantras to help keep your words and thoughts positive.

You read the *yamas* and the *niyamas* of yogic living earlier, and you may have already decided which ones reflect your general behavior best. Yoga uses ten very specific intentions: five negative social behaviors and five positive personal behaviors. I will show you how these intentions adapt to reflect birthing behaviors. You will choose one or two that will reflect how you want to behave during labor. Your choices become your meditation for managing your emotions while you work with your physical body. By choosing an intention that resonates with how you perceive your social behavior, you are more likely to stick to those intentions as your labor becomes increasingly intense.

Choosing your intention takes time and should be discussed with your birth partner. We will cover these birth intentions in detail in this chapter. There is a good chance that your partner knows you best and may even have some insight that you do not notice. They may be able to give you some perspective into your social behavior. I enjoy watching couples in my birthing classes discuss their birth intentions. When couples see their behaviors differently, it inevitably leads to some tension and mild arguing. I ask them to embrace the intention choosing process, really listen to each other's feedback, and deal with it now or at least before labor begins. If they are having a heated argument now, they will spare themselves the argument during labor.

As a birth coach, I tend to see situations arise such as these in labor:

Mom: Can you please be more attentive when I'm having a contraction? I feel like you don't care.

Partner: What do you want me to do? Every time I
try to touch you, you tell me to go away. So do it by
yourself.

In this particular instance, the mom has a tendency to be possessive or independent and doesn't easily welcome support even though she may really want it. This makes it difficult for her partner to understand how to support her. By taking the time to discuss their behavioral traits beforehand, this couple could decide that mom has a tendency to be possessive by nature. During labor, when Mom is showing possessive signs, her partner has the ability to remind her that she is regressing into a negative state by using their birth intention, which they set as being mindful of possessive behavior.

Or:

Mom: Please don't leave the room again—every time
you leave my sight, I feel worse and the contractions
are more painful.

Partner: But honey, I have to get you water so you
don't dehydrate.

In this situation, Mom is overly needy and demanding. This makes her partner feel like he is not doing the right things for her. If Mom has a natural behavioral habit of needing attention, the couple may decide that non-stealing is a word that they will use. When she becomes overly needy, her partner can bring up the birth intention, and Mom will recognize that she is bringing a negative quality into her birth experience.

These behaviors don't just occur in labor. They exist prior to labor, and recognizing your behavior and what you consider good versus negative action can become the conversation that you and your birth partner have in order to set the right intentions for your birth experience. Once you commit to your intention, it becomes the foundation for your labor. It will naturally set the foundation for a calm and meditative environment for the entire process. Your partner will be able to use your intentions as their method of motivation with you during difficult moments in labor.

These intentions become your reminders when you are starting to lose focus or feel like disconnecting from the experience. Since your intentions have been chosen based on your ideal birth and your personality, they will have a powerful effect on how you manage your emotions. When I am with a client in labor, I am amazed at how well they respond to their intentions. I use them as tools for focus and to help keep my client aware of what she is experiencing. When she becomes overwhelmed and seems to be giving in to pain, I repeat her intention and she immediately calms down and identifies with her behavior.

Here are your intentions for a yoga birth. I have included scenarios with each *yama* and *niyama* to help you understand how this particular intention works in labor. There are many different scenarios that can happen. You need to be creative in deciding your own scenarios for choosing the best intention for your birth plan.

Step 1: Intent to Refrain from Negative Behavior— Choosing a Yama

Step 1 requires you to set an intention to manage negative behavior in childbirth. These *yamas* can occur during moments of intense pain and frustration. Think about how you deal with difficulty on an everyday basis, and ask yourself if it were possible you would behave this way during labor. If you notice a behavioral *yama* trait that might be similar to your behavior, then that *yama* would be your birth intention.

Once you have read through them, take some time to reflect on their meaning and how they relate to you and your ideal birth. Discuss them with your partner and choose one that you both feel has the potential of appearing in labor. This will be your point of focus and your partner's tool for managing your motivation when you are creating a negative atmosphere.

Emotions from *yama* behaviors can cause tension and stress in the body. In labor, tension and stress restrict contractions, slow the dilation process, and cause shallow breathing.

As you read through the *yamas* for labor, you may find multiple examples that reflect how you might feel or act. Try to identify with just one or two. If you set too many intentions, you will lose focus, and none of them will work.

The negative behaviors (which in yoga are presented in the positive for emphasis) are:

- Nonviolence (*Ahimsa*)

- Truthfulness (*Satya*)

- Non-Stealing (*Asteya*)

- Moderation (*Brahmacharya*)

- Nonpossessiveness (*Aparigraha*)

Nonviolence

Nonviolence means managing aggression. When you feel pain or experience discomfort in any way, do you project your emotions aggressively toward others? Do you speak with anger and resentment toward yourself? Aggression can appear in labor as a coping strategy for pain, especially in active or transition stages. If you have had very little sleep and exhaustion is a battle for you, then you may start to behave in a manner that hurts others and takes you further into anger and pain. *Ahimsa* means you avoid lashing out at those around you, who only want the best for you and the baby. You must remain focused on the good intentions for your birth. When you reach a point of intolerable pain, it is possible to lose self-control. Once you have lost control, it is very hard to get it back. It becomes a waste of energy. You need to be aware of the feelings of others who are there to help you. You also need to be aware of your baby. The baby is hard at work in labor and needs you to create a nonaggressive atmosphere. The baby needs your support as they use your body through the birthing process.

> **Scenario:** Betty has been in labor for fifteen hours and has had no sleep. Her partner is also tired. He tries to comfort her by massaging her back, and she pushes him away. She says, "Don't touch me. Go away and leave me alone." Dad now has the ability to remind Mom that her words are harsh and go against their wishes of refraining from aggression.

Truthfulness

Truthfulness represents a vast amount of emotions in labor—how you project your words in negative self-talk, how you believe you can cope, what you are letting those around you think about how you feel. If you speak from a negative perspective or allow yourself to feel like you don't have the strength to manage pain, then you are manifesting your own negative birth story. Saying things like *I can't do this, this is way too painful, I just want a cesarean section,* or *I need medication* are powerful, and if you repeat them enough times in labor, you will believe them. You need to control your words in childbirth and be sincere in your actions. When you spend your energy on negativity, you give your body the cues it needs to give up. You also begin to self-destruct emotionally. Your support team will need to spend their energy talking you out of your beliefs. Be true to yourself. Say only what you mean, and try speaking with words of encouragement and strength. Your baby can hear you. Use nurturing words that promote a safe and wonderful birth.

> **Scenario:** Julie has been in labor for four hours and has been coping very well. She just had her cervix checked. She is three centimeters dilated. She becomes

discouraged and starts to tell her partner she can't take the pain anymore and that she can't keep going naturally. In this situation, by choosing truthfulness as their birth intention, her partner is able to remind her that discouraging words are not part of their plan and encourage her to speak in positive words.

Non-Stealing

Pain can be frightening when it is unknown and unmanaged. How do you manage pain generally? When you have the flu or a cold, do you tend to become needy and demanding? This needy behavior in labor drains the physical and emotional energy from your support team. When you become high maintenance, you exhaust everyone around you in a negative way. This is considered stealing energy from others. You have to trust your ability to cope. Your support team is there to help you manage pain and create comfort for you. Embrace what they have to offer without being selfish. You have to respect others and the role they play. When your baby is born, you will inevitably be tired and need rest. Your support team can help you with aftercare effectively if you allow them proper rest while balancing your care during labor.

> **Scenario:** Tania has been in labor for six hours and isn't managing her pain very well. She keeps asking for water, food, and for her back to be rubbed. Along with her partner, her mother is also there to support her. Her partner would like to take a nap to regain some energy while her mother steps in. Tania becomes upset and begs him to stay with her. In this situation, her need forattention prevents her support team from fully being able to assist her. By reminding her of this intention, she remembers how important it is to manage her time and her support team's time.

Moderation

Moderation represents patience and balance. You must be prepared for the natural birth experience without obsessing about the details. Cultivate the discipline for patience and allow an opportunity to surpass your pain threshold. Worrying about details that are not in the moment—such as what will happen next or how many more hours there are to go—takes away from each contraction as it happens. You take two steps back when you are obsessing about the ten steps ahead. Each contraction is vital to the cardinal movements your baby has to make and to the changes your cervix needs to make. Be present to the moment, and allow yourself to balance obsessive behavior with patience. Worrying about what's next is a normal emotion, but mindfulness of moderation eliminates panic and stress. It is okay to plan your coping strategy for the next phase of contractions and build your pain threshold, but there is no need to fret over how you will manage. Be in control of where you are now, and trust your plan to get to the last stage as it unfolds.

> **Scenario:** Michelle has been in labor for ten hours and has not stopped asking how much longer. She keeps asking when transition will happen. Each contraction, she starts to panic and worry about how long it will last. This prevents her from breathing properly and causes her contractions to feel worse than they would have otherwise. By reminding Michelle of her intention of moderation, she can calm herself and recognize that being in the moment is important to managing pain and focusing on the task at hand.

Nonpossessiveness

Nonpossessiveness means to embrace your experience with others and let go of your ego. Share the experience with your labor support team. They are there to help you through this wonderful experience. Allow them to be a part of your natural process as opposed to feeling like you need to manage it all by yourself. Abandon the notion that you own your experience and your baby. Being possessive will cause you to feel like you need to fight for what is yours. When you experience the negative energy of protection, you cause stress and anxiety in your body, which will put you in self-defense mode. Let it go.

Be open to allowing your birth experience to be shared. Your partner is equally entitled to experiencing the baby's birth. Your support team will share your birth story when it is over. You play a major part in making everyone's story wonderful when it is told. You do not need to micromanage your experience and make it a "me, me, me" story. Let your baby feel the energy of everyone around you. Surround yourself with security and love.

> **Scenario:** Christina has been in labor for two hours and is starting to show signs of exhaustion. It is 3 **am** and she has not had any sleep since the night before. Her partner suggests different positions to help her get some rest. She tells her partner to go to bed and let her do this alone. She said she is fine and can manage the contractions without any help. In this situation, her partner is able to remind her that he or she would like to be a part of the process and that nonpossessiveness was an intention they had set together.

Step 2: Intent to Practice Positivity— Choosing a Niyama

Step 2 is to set the intention of making your labor a positive experience. The *niyamas* give a clear description of what is considered positive behavior. This birth intention will become your most powerful tool for managing natural birth. *Niyamas* cultivate an awareness of patience, peace, and self-respect.

The intention that you choose will be the foundation of your birth story. It sets the tone for how you want your labor to unfold. As we eliminate negative behavior with *yamas*, we embrace the emotions and actions encouraged by *niyamas*. By being mindful of positive behavior, you naturally manifest a positive experience. The *niyamas* represent you. They give you the inspiration to directly connect your physical and spiritual well-being to your birth. They help you channel your energy toward your baby and create a sense of togetherness. As you read through them, try to visualize how that *niyama* shows itself in your situation. If the words stir a positive feeling in you, then that *niyama* may be the energy you would like to use within your birth. They are all wonderful behaviors. Remember to only choose one or two. If you have too many to focus on, then none of them will work.

The positive behaviors are:

- Purity (*Saucha*)
- Contentment (*Samtosha*)
- Discipline (*Tapas*)
- Self-Study (*Svadhyaya*)
- Divine Empowerment (*Ishvara Pranidhana*)

Purity

Purity embraces the wholeness of birth. Your body is a channel of energy that experiences the pain of labor, but that pain just passes through you, you do not have to own it. When you experience pain you need to respect your body, not push it away. Purity means to embrace each contraction as a means to bringing your baby closer to your arms. Each contraction has a job: to take baby through cardinal movements. By working with each contraction to maximize its purpose, you manage to stay present and allow yourself the ability to stay in control. Allow the pain to be your reminder of something wonderful you are experiencing, not something hurtful. Replace discomfort with love and respect, and use purity as the light in the tunnel of new life within you moving toward the world.

> **Scenario:** Jackie has been in labor for seven hours and feels like her contractions are starting to come closer together. She is definitely progressing to an active phase. She has been managing the intensity by visualizing her body opening up in each contraction and embracing a light that attaches to her breath. She keeps her breath calm and her energy pure in her body, which helps her baby along.

Contentment

Contentment means acceptance. As you read this and other books about labor, you are embracing birth education. You are becoming aware of the birthing process. When you are aware, you can make knowledgeable choices. The ability to make choices eliminates the fear of the unknown. You learn to accept your circumstances as they unfold. Practicing contentment in labor gives you the power to accept things as they happen. Trust your knowledge, and be present to each moment. Don't worry over what might happen or if the choices you are making are wrong. Go with the flow and be open to your birth experience. Labor with confidence, and know deep within that you are in control and aware of everything as it is in the moment.

Scenario: Lisa has been in labor for nine hours and is at six centimeters dilated. She hasn't dilated past that in over two hours. She has been offered Pitocin to help encourage dilation. She decides to turn down the Pitocin and trust that if she tries more postures she can encourage her baby to descend and dilate. She asks for more time to work on her own.

Discipline

Discipline represents your birth plan before you start labor. If you are choosing an unmedicated birth, then it may require discipline to get through the times when contraction intensity increases. If you struggle with willpower generally, then discipline will be a challenge in labor. However, being mindful of discipline as your birth intention will keep your willpower at the forefront of your decisions. If you are being offered an epidural by the medical staff, it takes a lot of discipline to turn it down. Being aware of your choices and managing them as you make them requires the discipline to believe in your birth plan. If you want a natural birth, then stay committed to it. Trust the strength of your body and your ability to use the YBM techniques as you work through those difficult moments.

Scenario: Monica has been in active labor for four hours. She decides to go to the hospital since her contractions have been four minutes apart for the last two hours. She is eight centimeters dilated and admitted to the hospital. She is offered an epidural and told she may not have an opportunity later. She is in pain and an epidural seems enticing so she can get some rest. She decides she is almost there and wants to manage her contractions on her own.

Self-Study

Childbirth can teach you many things about your strengths and weaknesses. When you direct the mind and body through contractions, you discover your inner strength. Labor is a passage into self-discovery that only a woman is given as a gift to experience. Allow childbirth to be your teacher. Learn about yourself through the stages of pain management. Your emotions and reactions can be your best resource for personal growth. Self-study in labor manifests presence and awareness. You take responsibility for everything you do. You are awake to everything you feel as you become observant to how you manage this very important time in your life.

> **Scenario:** Sophia has been in labor for fifteen hours. She is tired but has managed her pain very well. She is amazed at her own strength. She was sure that she had no pain tolerance and would need an epidural. She has been using her postures and really emphasizing her breath in each phase. With every contraction, she relies on feeling stronger and more in control rather than believing she wasn't going to be able to last.

Divine Empowerment

Divine empowerment is something beyond you. There is a source of energy, and whether it is God, a higher power, or the universe, it oversees all things. This divine energy senses your needs and desires. By choosing a natural birth and allowing divine energy to guide you there, you surrender to the power of your soul to birth with faith and trust. By connecting with divine energy during labor, you invite peace and serenity in your birthing experience.

> **Scenario:** Diane has just started labor an hour ago and feels like the contractions are unmanageable. She recognizes that this is the beginning and asks her god to help her build tolerance. She allows her faith to manage

her pain tolerance. After each contraction, she thanks her god silently and trusts that he will give her the strength to manage the next one.

Once you have chosen your intentions, you are ready to connect them to your physical experience of birth. This physical experience occurs in the body, and learning how to work with your body through contractions is your tool of application toward labor progression.

Step 3: Awareness of the Body— Using Postures During Labor

Asanas, or postures, encourage the physical work of labor. They help you connect with your body as opposed to disassociate from it. Since labor is an experience of body, you don't want to let contractions take over. You want to guide contractions through your body and work with them to help the baby descend. Postures are considered mindful movement exercises that encourage physical freedom. Your intentions help keep your thoughts directed to your labor experience and allow the body to open in each of the laboring stages. As you may feel pain from contractions, postures are used to help you go deeper into the pain to encourage dilation of the cervix and the cardinal movements of your baby.

The YBM *asanas* are specific tools to work with progression. Following the specific posture sequences (sometimes called a flow) and postures for each stage enables you to control your body. This enhances the progression of contractions and speeds the dilation and effacement process.

Each phase in the first stage of labor has an *asana* sequence you will follow. You only need to know these specific postures in the yoga system. Even though yoga incorporates over 500 postures, for the purpose of labor, only the few poses outlined here are effective in labor. You can practice the early sequence anywhere in your pregnancy as an excellent way to prepare for labor.

I have chosen these laboring postures for many reasons. They are similar to comfort measures already used by doulas and midwives, and they target muscle groups in the body that relieve pelvic pressure, encourage efficient labor, and help make the pushing stage easier.

These postures have a direct correlation to how the body works in labor. By working through these *asanas*, you work directly with the baby—in other words, you use your body to make cardinal movements easier for the baby. You help prevent posterior positioning and encourage vertex anterior positioning. You let the baby know that you are there and trying to make their work easier.

The postures are broken down by phase of labor: early, active, and transition. You will be following the posture sequences while you are in that phase of labor. It is difficult to know where your cervix is in the dilation process, but, as we covered earlier, you will have some idea of where you are just by how your body is responding to the emotional signs. These *asanas* will be explained for each phase in detail in the next chapter.

The early labor sequence consists of the following poses, which you would do as a flow from one pose to the next:

- Child's
- Cat/Cow
- Downward Dog
- Squat
- Mountain
- Warrior II
- Triangle
- Wide-Angle Forward Bend
- Pigeon
- Crescent Lunge

- Frog
- Butterfly

Doing these poses in sequence keeps the muscles stretching and allows the body to go deep into opening. By moving through flow you also encourage yourself to keep active, which is really important in labor. Lying on your back slows labor down and makes it more painful. When you lie on your back, you make it harder for the baby to find space to make movements; in addition, when you are reclined it is difficult for baby to descend over the coccyx bone, the end of the spine that we know as the tailbone.

When you stay in one position through labor, you become vulnerable to the pain without having a way to work with it. One of the things I stress in prenatal yoga classes is the freedom of mobility. Using the flow of postures allows you to experience mobility and enables you to keep the body limber and able to manage the change of poses when pain becomes almost unbearable. Teaching yourself to flow in early labor will give you the strength you need to move in transition when you will have the most resistance to movement.

The active labor postures consist of seven postures that were part of the early flow:

- Child's
- Cat/Cow
- Squat
- Mountain
- Wide-Angle Forward Bend
- Crescent Lunge
- Frog

Active labor is more intense then early labor, and contractions are a little closer together. This makes it harder to do all of the early flow postures. Exhaustion and discomfort limits your ability to flow through all the poses with ease. Therefore, using the seven poses one at a time over several contractions will still give you the benefit of promoting dilation with each contraction.

Active labor will be your first hurdle to managing without medication. You will be in what is considered "good" labor because at this phase you should be over four centimeters and progressing to stronger contractions. Rather than flow, you would now hold your *asanas* as laboring positions. This will help your support team also give you some comfort, as I will discuss in some hands-on tips in the next chapter. The idea is to use all seven postures in active labor but at a much slower and more stable pace to manage each contraction individually. By doing this, you are still considered mobile and you are able to remain in control and present in the moment. As you hold each pose, you allow yourself to focus on breathing and your birthing intention.

Once you come into transition—at approximately eight centimeters—you will be very limited physically. As we discussed earlier, transition will feel the hardest on your body physically and challenge you the most emotionally. The physical changes to your body are intense as your baby moves into the smaller diameter of the pelvis and creates pressure on your bowels and nerves. Moving can feel almost impossible and unbearable as you realize each contraction gets more intense with movement. In this phase, women tend to find a position and cocoon themselves away from the world. You will rely on your support team the most in this phase to keep you on the right track and to prevent you from withdrawing.

In transition we use three postures that are crucial to keeping this phase as short as possible:

- Cat/Cow

- Squat

- Child's

You may start to struggle between continuing naturally and relieving your pain with an epidural. Try to focus on your intention. The Yoga Birth Method manages your body by using postures that reflect the most natural ways to position it for birth or for the next stage, which is pushing.

As we work the *asanas*, the next step in the pathway goes hand in hand with movement. Breathing is the most important part of natural labor, and it can make a difference in how you control your emotions and stay connected to your birth experience.

Step 4: Breath (Pranayama)— The Link Between Mind and Body

Life is breath. It is as simple as that statement. Everything we do requires us to breathe. If there is no breath, there can be no life— yet we take our breath for granted.

How often do you stop and say, "Wow, I am breathing!" If you did that a few times a day, you can imagine how much presence you would bring to your life on a daily basis. How you breathe reflects how you live. When your breath is shallow and fast, it means you are stressed and anxious. When your breath is short and stays in your chest, it means you are impatient. Fast, deep breathing reflects anger and anxiety. All the signs are there if you just stop and watch your breath. If you take a moment to diagnose your breath, you will be able to truly diagnose your emotions and your well-being.

Breath is vital to labor. It makes the difference between a stressed and anxious birth and a calm and patient birth. If we removed the eight-step pathway and all other birthing options available and had you focus on your breathing in labor, you could probably manage the entire birth naturally. This is why other birthing techniques focus on breath alone. However, keep in mind that breathing the right way in labor does not guarantee a natural birth, because there are so many other obstacles in the way, such as what you're feeling physically and

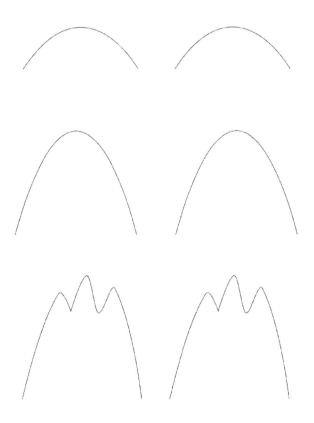

how your ego plays tricks on you emotionally. This is why the YBM is so powerful and effective in accomplishing an unmedicated birth. It addresses all the obstacles and uses breath as a link to managing those obstacles.

In the YBM we manage pain by managing breath. In the same way we changed our postures in each phase of labor, we will also change our breathing technique. Your breathing will also take on the *Om* sound. *Om* is a universal sound that connects inner energy to the energy around you. By concentrating on hearing the *Om* at the back of the throat, it calms the body and brings awareness to the work of your breath.

Practice this *Om* breath: sit comfortably and take a few deep breaths. When you are ready, on your next deep exhalation, push your breath out through the mouth and add the sound *Om* as long as you can.

When the intensity of contractions change, the way we breathe through that intensity must also change. Contractions are typically explained by comparing mountain elevations.

In early labor (top), your contractions will feel like a mole hill. They will be short, between 30 and 45 seconds, and the peak will fade quickly.

In active labor (middle), your contractions will feel like climbing a steeper hill. They will be longer, between 45 and 90 seconds, and the peak will feel more intense at the top.

In transition (bottom), your contractions will come without many breaks in between and feel like multiple peaks at the top. They will last 60 to 90 seconds and feel as if they don't end.

During delivery, the last breathing technique you will use is called *Sukha Purvaka*. We will cover this in detail in chapter 6.

It is impossible to breathe through each phase of contractions the same way, because they require different coping strategies. If you try to use the same breath for each phase, you will lose the ability to manage the peaks. This is one reason why most birthing techniques fail during active labor. When you are experiencing a different feeling of pain than a few hours prior, how can the same tool work? The YBM gives you three different breathing techniques that help you manage the elevation level of pain as it increases.

In early labor, use *Ujjayi* breath. This is also called ocean breathing in yoga. It is the preferred breath during yoga practice because it calms the nervous system and helps relax the body. Deep ocean breathing allows the body to go deeper into the pose, as the breath is full and calm. In labor, ocean breathing helps you stay connected to what you are feeling and encourages you to come into a state of calm relaxation. As intensity increases, the sound of the *Om* can be vocalized. As you work through the smaller mountains of contractions, ocean breathing and silent *Oms* help to manage the time and length of contractions while enabling your body to dilate and labor to progress into active phase.

When you move into active labor, things will change. Your contractions will be closer together and stronger. You may be tired or frustrated. *Ujjayi* breathing will not be strong enough to carry you through the intensity of contractions. In active labor, when we start to see changes in emotions, we make the first adjustment by changing the breathing. We start to use *Dirga* breathing, or elevator breathing, and visualize longer *Oms*. *Dirga* is similar to *Ujjayi* breathing except the inhale and the exhale are extended to a full count of three. Rather than breathing in and out at an even pace, you breathe in while visualizing an elevator rising three floors. When you exhale, you visualize the descent into the abdomen as if the elevator is moving dowm. It is one long, continuous breath managed with the count of three in and three out. Your support person can also help to keep you focused and in control during this stage by managing the count as you breathe. By having your support person count *in…two…three…out…two… three,* it will keep you on track to managing pain and being in the present moment.

As you manage progression using postures and breath, you will find that you come into the yogini groove. In active labor, as you use the YBM techniques, you should be able to get through this phase calmly and fully focused on being present. In difficult moments, remember that this method provides you with the tools and techniques you need to guide you through those moments. Using the techniques will take the edge off emotionally and allow you to manage your contractions from a state of grace and acceptance.

As you progress naturally, you will soon come into the transition phase. This is your final hurdle before pushing begins. The amazing part of getting through labor naturally is that this stage will pass quickly if the body is unmedicated. Keep in mind, it is also at this stage where you may feel the strongest need to take medication. Sometimes you may even be dealing with a posterior baby and slow progression, and the best thing to do is take an epidural to help manage the setbacks that are not in your control. As we discussed earlier, when you come into transition, you will immediately recognize the intense physical signs that you're feeling. When you start to feel overwhelmed physically with pressure from your baby's head and the intensity of frequent contractions, the slow-paced deep breathing will not be enough to sustain patience through the intensity of contractions that are very close together. At this point, you would introduce *Kapalbhati* breath, or fire breathing. This breathing technique for labor is modified from the full yogic version. In this breath, you take a deep inhalation and then push three or four exhales from the mouth. In this phase, women tend to naturally start breathing from the mouth. However, when they are not mindful of breath, then pushing air out from the mouth without an inhalation gets very exhausting and drains energy. It also causes stress and anxiety. Women will start to breathe in a panicked manner and make loud *hee hee hee* and *ooooohhh ouuuuhh* sounds. Some women tend to scream and yell in this stage, as opposed to keeping their breathing under control. *Kapalbhati* is the perfect breath here, as it addresses the natural breath and sounds that you would use without guidance. The key to *Kapalbhati* is to ensure that for every three or four exhalations there is one deep inhalation. The mindfulness of that one inhalation makes a world of difference toward how you manage to maintain awareness and control.

Once you reach ten centimeter's dilation and 100 percent effacement in transition, you are ready to work the second stage of labor—pushing. The breathing in this stage is a ten-count hold breath. This breath must be directed to the perineum muscle in order to push baby out efficiently. Sometimes, women hold their breath but let air escape upward or don't use their power in a downward direction. This is called purple pushing. To push your baby out, you must bear down and push the breath internally downward for a full count of ten at least four times in one contraction. Typically, most hospitals use this ten-count hold breath. It may be different if you use a midwife or give birth at a hospital using a more natural approach to pushing. In the YBM we use *Sukha Purvaka* (see page 178) to make this breathing stage as natural as possible. I love this natural approach to pushing; it makes this stage calmer and more controlled by the mother as opposed to a medically directed delivery. When you are in labor and you reach the pushing stage, you may want to discuss with your practitioners and nursing staff your desire to avoid the counting in the room and allow you to manage your pushing on your own. As we go into the application details for the YBM in the next three chapters, we will discuss the entire how-to of each breath as it relates to labor.

Let's Review:
- Early Labor—Ocean Breath (*Ujjayi*)
- Active Labor—Three-Part Breath (*Dirga*)
- Transition—Fire Breath (*Kapalbhati*)
- Pushing—Count/Hold Breath (*Sukha Purvaka*)

The first four steps along the pathway are hands-on, and when you practice them simultaneously in labor they naturally lead you into the remaining steps. The last four steps are the results of using the YBM. They create a calm, mindful, and enlightened childbirth experience without forcing the outcome. Once you have applied steps 1 through 4, you will notice the next steps become your demeanor in labor.

Step 5: Pratyahara, or Sense Withdrawal— Surrender to the Natural Process

Intention, *asana* practice, and breathing are the techniques that will help manage pain and encourage progression. When you surrender to your birth intention, breath, and posture practice, you bring yourself to a state of acceptance and presence that allows you to be fully connected to what is happening to you. You may still feel pain in contractions, but your coping mechanism will be calmer and more peaceful. Surrender means to trust the YBM technique to help you achieve natural birth. You will have no expectations or fear. You will be in the experience of bringing your child to the world as opposed to being in pain.

Sense withdrawal is release from physical pain. When you go into labor thinking pain is being done to you, you will fight it and try to get away from it. Sense withdrawal in yoga practice is to be led by inner energy, breath, and movement, not by ego. The principle of sense withdrawal is that all things you see or feel externally do not make up who you are. Being present to your energy and being aware of your inner self are what make up who you are. This is true to labor. As you connect to your pain from a deeper level within you, be present to the energy of the labor process. Let go of whatever comes up emotionally that seems difficult and surrender to what is happening as it unfolds. Don't allow external distractions to control your birthing process. Trust in your natural ability to give birth to your child. As we apply the techniques, you will learn how to turn off sensory distractions that come up in labor.

Step 6: Concentration (Dharana)—Mindful Connections to Contractions

As labor progresses, exhaustion and frustration can lead to choosing pain medications and medical assistance. Work though natural labor one step at a time. You have been given the tools to do that in this birthing method. You will find that as you use the tools, you have a direct focus. You do not need to keep reminding yourself to be calm or to be present. You will do that without force because you are mindful of following the YBM pathway. As each contraction happens, you have a plan and the resources to get through it. Mindfulness happens as you are present to breath, movement, and your intention.

If you face a roadblock, you have the ability to use a different posture, change your breath, and even use a different intention that is more helpful. Being in a state of mindfulness is what all birthing techniques try to accomplish, but they ask you to remind yourself of it constantly. The YBM takes you into it as you flow, breathe, and embody your intention throughout labor. When you are mindful, you are capable of recognizing options or decisions that might need to be made in labor and, most importantly, help you to avoid medication as a coping strategy. You become fully aware of how each contraction is a milestone to bringing baby closer to your arms.

You can also use the mantras in chapter 2. Mantras are powerful sentences that provide a direct focus. They are words that give you reminders to remain positive, calm, and peaceful. When things are difficult or you feel frustrated, a mantra can help change your thinking pattern and replace negative thoughts. If one or a few of the mantras resonate with you and fit into your birth intention, then take it into your birth. Repeat it as many times as you feel you need to; allow the mantra to embody your breath, body, and mind.

Step 7: Meditation (Dhyana)—Embracing a Calm State in Labor

By using these steps as the pathway of labor, you mindfully embrace the feeling of calmness and inner strength. The YMB pathway is an uninterrupted flow of concentration aimed to heighten the blissful experience of labor and create oneness with the universe. When you progress through the three stages of labor committed to your intention and deeply connected to breath and body, you are in a state of natural meditation. This calm state invites the baby to trust your body during the birthing process. This trusting relationship between you and your baby reduces the chances of dystocia and medical intervention.

Meditation is difficult when it is expected or planned. It should be a state of energy that embraces you when you breathe and move. The YBM invites this energy in without force because the mind, body, and spirit are in harmony through breath control, body movement, and thought focus. Meditation does not have to be a "sitting still" experience—there are many ways to bring mediation into practice. The YBM is a movement of meditation that creates an enlightened experience.

Step 8: Experiencing Relationship (Samadhi)

The ultimate goal of the eight-step pathway is the realization that you and your child have been brought together by the power of the universe. It is a state of peace, completion, compassion, and selfless love.

By committing to an enlightened birth experience, you embody a strength that encourages you through the natural process. You accomplish enlightenment when your child is born. You will open your heart with love that is unconditional. You bear a responsibility for the soul that has come into your life. The joy of holding your child for the first time brings bliss instantly. It is unconditional, selfless love that makes the entire process of labor worth it.

You have now connected all eight steps of the pathway to your labor. You will achieve mindfulness through intention, connection through body movement, and calmness through breath. Surrender keeps you in the experience of labor and in the present moment. You are laboring with a mindfulness that creates a deep meditative state. The end brings enlightenment: holding your child for the first time.

April's Birth Story

My pregnancy with Guinevere was more challenging than my other three. It was challenging not so much on a physical level but on emotional, psychological, and spiritual levels. The challenges were all blessings, of course, because they allowed me to learn more about myself and grow so much as a mother, wife, and woman.

From the beginning of the pregnancy, I felt her spirit; it was very gentle, peaceful, and full of love. My little girl even made herself known to many of us by visiting in dreams. I had no doubt that she was a special soul who had picked us as her family. I felt that this birthing would be spiritual for me, and that once she was here, she would just fit right in like she belonged here.

My doula suggested The Yoga Birth Method. As an avid lover of yoga, I ordered the book right away, expecting some wonderful positions to help me through my pregnancy and birth. When I got the book, I breezed through it and immediately found peace in the postures for the second trimester (Frog was my absolute favorite!). But what I really enjoyed the most was working through the questions it asked. It was through reading this book that I realized I had made myself a victim during my first birth. This may not sound like a big revelation, but to me it meant everything. I saw how I had made myself a victim not only in my first birth but during other hard times in my life as well. It was then and there that I vowed to make this birthing different.

Nearing the end of my pregnancy, I would do my third-trimester postures and soon found which ones I knew I would use the most in labor. I had talks with my doula and others who would be at the birth, telling them what postures I enjoyed the most and to remind me to use them. I also told them about my revelation and to never allow me to go to that place during labor.

One Saturday I started feeling light contractions. I didn't pay much attention to them because I frequently felt contractions in the evening.

Sunday morning I went out for brunch. Throughout the day I was feeling contractions, and around dinnertime, I knew that they weren't stopping: this was it. I used some of the early labor postures from the Yoga Birth Method book, and many of them made me feel so good—I really enjoyed anything that opened my hips. I was getting a bit frustrated that contractions wouldn't get closer together. They were about ten minutes apart, very consistently. Around 6 am, I decided to eat and gain some energy. My labor progressed throughout the day.

Finally, I was sitting backwards on the downstairs toilet, because this felt amazing—it was just like the squat I learned in the Yoga Birth

Method and totally opened up my hips. It was dark in the room, with just a few candles lit. This is when I had my emotional release and sobbed like a child. I felt like nothing was happening despite my best efforts. I was scared that I couldn't do it for as long as I would need to, but most of all, I think I just needed to sob like a baby. It was such a release for me. This was different than me feeling like a victim like before — this was me relinquishing control. It was a huge step for me.

I went downstairs to the tub. Steve, my husband, got in with me, although instead of resting on him I was on my knees, leaning over the side of the tub. Things were very intense at this point. I started vomiting and knew I must be close. I reached up inside and felt her head — she was up there, but not too far. I wanted to see what would happen if I pushed, so for the next contraction I pushed when I felt the urge and was really surprised when her head came all the way to the opening of my vagina. With the next contraction, I pushed her head out to about her brow line. I stopped because it hurt!

I decided that I had to keep pushing because, well, what else could I do? So with the next contraction I pushed with all my might while touching her head the whole time, and I felt her head just pop out. Without even thinking I pushed with all my might again; I wanted to meet my baby. In an instant she was out! I did it! I pushed her out into Steve's hands. He was the first to hold our sweet little girl.

Guinevere was born peacefully at home, surrounded by so much love. She nursed like a pro within twenty minutes of being born. The Yoga Birth Method helped me achieve this without medication, enabling Guinevere to be fully alert.

6

It's Yoga Birth Time!

This chapter is your go-to chapter during labor. When you start to recognize the signs of labor, you can come directly to this section and start to apply the tools to get you into the yogini groove. This chapter is set up as a checklist for you to be able to identify your stage of labor by assessing your physical and emotional signs and then applying the YBM for that stage. As you experience contractions, use the checklists below. If you feel you have reached a new phase, then move to the next list and use those specific tools.

Early Labor Stage

Remember as you begin to experience pain that this is only the beginning. What have you decided to use as your birth intentions? Now is the time to embrace them.

As you begin the flow and start your breathing, your intention becomes your focus. Stay connected to it is as each negative thought comes over you. Your intention is your foundation for the rest of the tools to work.

In early labor, your goal is to help your body to dilate and efface past three centimeters in order to move into active labor or what is considered good labor by your doctor.

What's Happening?

Physical Signs

- My contractions have started—
  light cramping off and on.

- My contractions are coming anywhere
  from 15 to 40 minutes apart.

- My contractions feel manageable
  while walking and talking.

- My contractions are lasting anywhere
  from 15 to 45 seconds long.

- I am able to relax between contractions.

- It is the middle of the night; I should get some
  sleep and get ready for good labor to begin.

Emotional Signs

- I feel very excited and happy.

- I am aware of what I am going through
  and have embraced my intention.

- I feel talkative.

- I am trying to remain calm even though
  I realize my baby is coming.

- I feel some tension and worry, but I am mindful
  of my tools to manage this process.

Yoga Birth Method for Early Labor

Concentration/Meditation

- It is the start of labor. It is important for me to
  begin the practice of concentration/meditation
  by using my *asanas* and breathing techniques.

- The pain may seem difficult, but it is only the beginning and I am increasing my pain threshold.
- I have told the baby my birth intention, and we are committed to working together.

Breathing Technique

Ujjayi Breathing: Deep Ocean Breathing and Silent Om Exhalation

How to: Inhale deeply through the nose and exhale through the nose. On the exhale, feel the breath push on the back of the throat, creating a natural "Om wave" sound.

Purpose: *Ujjayi* breathing encourages deep abdominal relaxation, which will enable you to start labor from a calm state and help your body relax. *Ujjayi* breathing gives you a very focused approach to breath awareness and begins your state of meditation. *Ujjayi* triggers the relaxation response in the body and helps you cope with the first phase of contractions.

Yoga Postures

- Yoga postures will help advance labor progression to active phase, using gravity to assist baby's descent into the birth canal. Postures that encourage hip, inner thigh, and leg stretches will prepare the body for the "pressure" feeling in active/transition stage and pushing stage.
- Use this 15-minute routine between contractions and throughout the early phase hours.

- Your support person can assist with pillows, hot/cold therapy, massage techniques, and hands-on assistance in poses.

Early Stage Flow

Child's Pose

How it helps:
- Releases tension and stress and quiets the mind.

- Turns off external stimulus that provokes negative emotions.

- Allows time to invite awareness of labor.

- Opens the hips and inner thighs, stretches sacrum, prevents back labor.

Comfort measures:
- Use a birthing ball or pillows under the forehead.

- Rest upper body on a birthing ball and rock the hips up and down.

- Apply a hot water bottle or ice pack to the lower back.

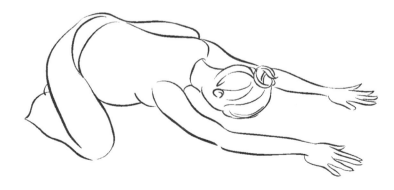

- Place pillows under the sit bones, which are the boney parts of your pelvis that you can feel on either side of your buttocks.

- Support person can press the space in the sacrum on either side of the spine to release contraction tension (called "sacrum squeeze").

How to do this pose:

- On your knees, touch your big toes together.

- Release your chest and head to the mat.

- Extend your arms outward and breathe deeply.

Cat Pose

How it helps:

- Removes tension throughout the vertebrae.

- Calms the central nervous system.

- Moves breath through the spine and into the contraction.

- Eases back pressure.

Comfort measures:

- Rest upper body on a birthing ball and roll the hips from side to side.

- Apply a hot water bottle or ice pack to the lower back.

- Support person can press the space in the sacrum on either side of the spine to release contraction tension (called "sacrum squeeze").

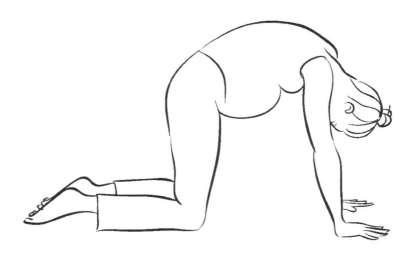

How to do this pose:

- On your hands and knees, assume Table Pose.

- On the inhalation, press into your hands and lift the belly button to your spine.

- Keep your hips in line with your knees.

- Breathe out to a neutral spine.

IT'S YOGA BIRTH TIME!

Cow Pose

How it helps:

- Removes tension throughout the vertebrae.

- Calms the central nervous system.

- Moves breath through the spine and into the contraction.

- Eases back tension.

Comfort measures:

- Rest upper body on a birthing ball and rock the hips up and down.

- Apply a hot water bottle or ice pack to the lower back.

- Support person can press the space in the sacrum on either side of the spine to release contraction tension (called "sacrum squeeze").

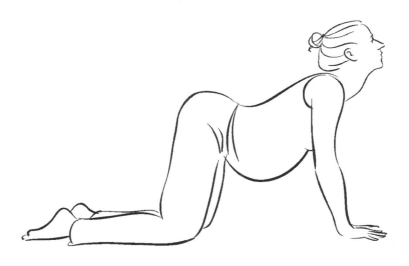

How to do this pose:

- On your hands and knees, breathe in, drop your belly toward the floor, and look up.

- Keep your hips in line with your spine.

- Exhale to neutral spine.

Downward Dog Pose

How it helps:

- Removes tension throughout the spine, shoulders, and neck.

- Increases oxygen to the placenta.

- Opens the sacrum and hips.

- Reduces fatigue.

- Eases back tension.

Comfort measures:

- Bend knees to release hamstrings.

- Use a chair or the side of a bed to raise upper body higher.

- Support person can press the space in the sacrum on either side of the spine to release contraction tension (called "sacrum squeeze").

- Support person can pull hips back and stretch spine further.

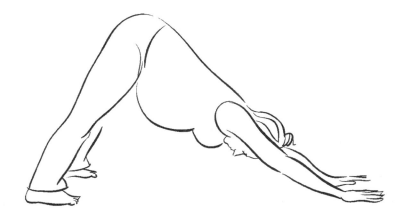

How to do this pose:

- On your hands and knees, curl your toes under and push into your hands to lift your tailbone up.

- Push into your hands and extend your spine.

- Stretch down through the legs. Bend your knees if your legs feel very tight.

- Take deep breaths.

Squat Pose

How it helps:

- Removes tension throughout the spine, shoulders, and neck.

- Increases oxygen to the placenta.

- Opens the sacrum and hips.

- Encourages dilation during contractions.

- Reduces fatigue.

- Eases back tension.

Comfort measures:

- Bend knees to release hamstrings.

- Use a chair or the side of a bed to raise upper body higher.

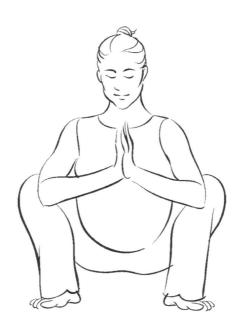

- Support person can assist squat from behind by holding arms.

- Support person can press the space in the sacrum on either side of the spine to release contraction tension (called "sacrum squeeze").

- Support person can pull hips back and stretch spine further.

- Ensure the spine is upright and straight.

How to do this pose:

- Stand with feet hip-distance apart.

- Bend the knees and lower yourself down to the floor.

- Keep the back straight and try not to sink into the hips.

- Support yourself with a birthing ball, wall, or partner if necessary.

- Keep your shoulders relaxed and breathe.

Mountain Pose

How it helps:

- Encourages gravity to bring baby into the birth canal.

- Helps baby maintain anterior vertex position.

- Helps breath move deep into abdomen.

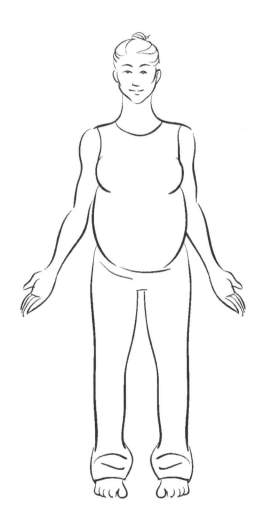

Comfort measures:

- Rock hips from side to side in a circular motion to help cardinal movements.

- Support person can press the space in the sacrum on either side of the spine to release contraction tension (called "sacrum squeeze").

- You and support person can slow dance to ease back tension.

How to do this pose:

- In a standing position, separate your feet slightly wider than hip-distance apart.

- Stand tall and lift your spine upward.

- Relax your shoulders and breathe deeply.

IT'S YOGA BIRTH TIME!

Warrior II Pose

How it helps:

- Removes tension throughout the spine, shoulders, and neck.

- Increases oxygen to the placenta.

- Opens the sacrum, inner thighs, and hips.

- Encourages a warriorlike attitude.

- Reduces fatigue.

- Eases back tension.

Comfort measures:

- Hands can stay on hips to ease shoulders.

- Support person can hold on to inner thighs from behind and encourage an external rotation.

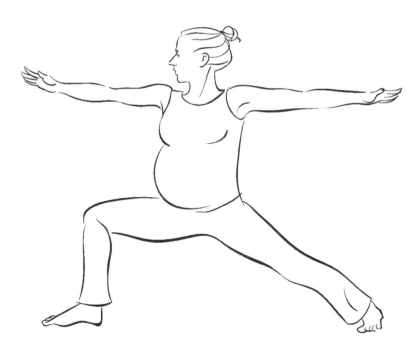

How to do this pose:

- Stand with your feet comfortably wide apart.

- Turn your back foot out 90 degrees and point your front foot forward.

- Make sure your heels are in line with each other.

- Bend the front knee over the ankle.

- Keep your spine straight and raise the arms to a T position.

- Look over your front hand and breathe deeply.

- Try to rotate your inner thighs out toward your little toes.

IT'S YOGA BIRTH TIME!

Triangle Pose

How it helps:

- Encourages baby to align with the birth canal.

- Opens the hips and inner thighs and gives baby space for internal rotation.

- Reduces fatigue.

- Eases back tension.

- Prepares hips and adductor muscles for pushing stage.

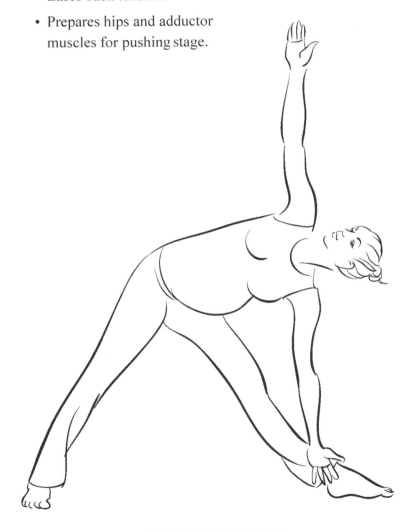

Comfort measures:

- Place bottom hand on a chair or yoga brick for stability.

- Support person can assist with hip opening by placing hands on top hip and encouraging a gentle stretch.

How to do this pose:

- Stand with your feet comfortably wide apart.

- Turn your back foot out 90 degrees and point your front foot forward.

- Make sure your heels are in line with each other and both your knees are straight.

- Lift your arms to a T position and extend your front hand over your toes.

- Release your front hand to your thigh or to the floor, whichever feels more comfortable.

- Open the hips and chest and raise your back arm upward.

- Breathe deeply.

Wide-Angle Forward Bend Pose

How it helps:

- Removes tension throughout the spine, lower back, and inner thighs.

- Increases oxygen to the placenta.

- Opens the sacrum and hips.

- Encourages baby to move into anterior position.

- Eases back labor.

Comfort measures:

- Bend knees to release hamstrings.

- Use a chair, side of a bed, or a wall to raise upper body higher.

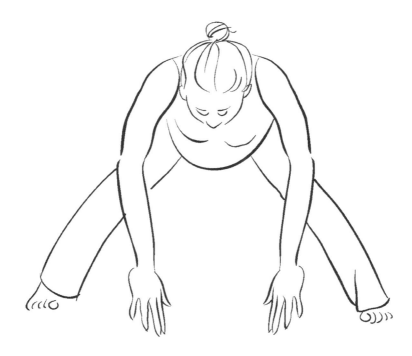

- Using a birthing ball, rock hips in a circular motion to help cardinal movements.

- Support person can press the space in the sacrum on either side of the spine to release contraction tension (called "sacrum squeeze").

- Support person can pull hips up to encourage baby's alignment into the birth canal.

How to do this pose:

- Stand with your legs wider than hip-distance apart.

- Straighten through the legs and extend forward from the hips.

- As you bend forward, try to keep your spine straight.

- Release your hands toward the floor. If you cannot touch the floor, place your hands on your shins or thighs.

- As you breathe, try to extend the spine and straighten the legs.

Pigeon Pose

How it helps:

- Encourages baby to align with the birth canal.

- Encourages dilation during contractions.

- Opens the hips and gives baby space for internal rotation.

- Prevents and relieves back labor/sciatica nerve.

- Prepares hips and adductor muscles for pushing stage.

Comfort measures:

- Rest upper body on pillow or birthing ball.

- Support person can assist with hip opening by placing hands on hips and encouraging a gentle stretch by pulling back.

- Apply a hot water bottle or ice pack to the lower back.

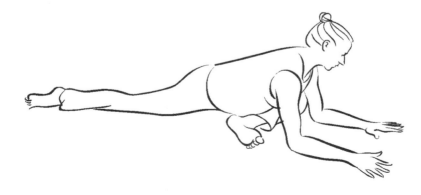

How to do this pose:

- On your hands and knees, slide one leg forward, drop the knee to the side, and extend the foot to the other side.

- Lower your hips over the bent leg and extend the straight leg further back.

- Release your head and shoulders as comfortably as you can. Use your elbows to manage your comfort level. As you become more flexible, you may find you can release your chest to the floor and extend your arms forward.

- Breathe deeply.

Crescent Lunge

How it helps:

- Encourages baby to align with the birth canal.

- Encourages dilation during contractions.

- Opens the hips and gives baby
  space for internal rotation.

- Prevents and relieves back labor.

- Prepares hips and adductor muscles for pushing stage.

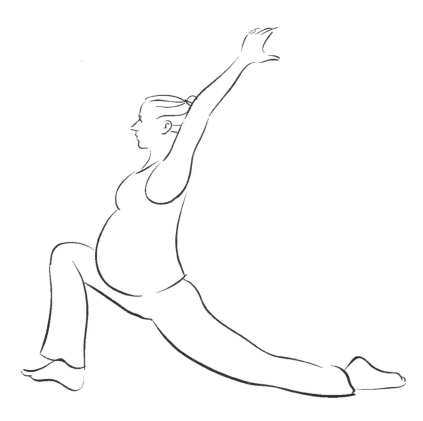

Comfort measures:

- Rest upper body on pillow or birthing ball.

- Support person can press the space in the sacrum on either side of the spine to release contraction tension (called "sacrum squeeze").

- Place pillows under back knee.

How to do this pose:

- On your knees, extend one leg out in front of you, foot flat on the floor, and bend into the leg until the knee reaches 90 degrees.

- Extend the other leg strongly backward.

- Lift the arms up and relax the shoulders.

- As you breathe, keep working into a lunge and focus on opening the chest.

Frog Pose

How it helps:

- Stretches the perineum.

- Stretches the muscles in the hips.

- Opens the inner thighs and hips.

- Encourages dilation during contractions.

Comfort measures:

- Place pillows under forehead.

- Support person can press the space in the sacrum on either side of the spine to release contraction tension (called "sacrum squeeze").

- Ensure feet are wider apart than knees.

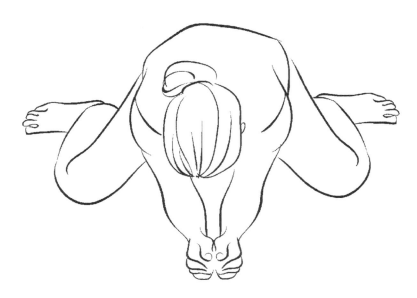

How to do this pose:

- On your hands and knees, move the knees wider than the hips.

- Bend your elbows to the floor.

- Extend the feet out wider than the knees and flex the toes up toward your face.

- Slightly push the tailbone back until you feel a deep stretch in the hips. Do not bounce in and out. Hold the stretch and allow your body to release.

- Breathe deeply.

IT'S YOGA BIRTH TIME!

Butterfly Pose

How it helps:

- Relaxes the entire body.

- Increases oxygen to the placenta.

- Opens the inner thighs and hips.

- Encourages dilation during contractions.

- Helps baby descend into the birth canal.

Comfort measures:

- Sit on a pillow to lift up hips and help baby align.

- Support person can assist squat from behind by holding arms.

- Ensure the spine is upright and straight.

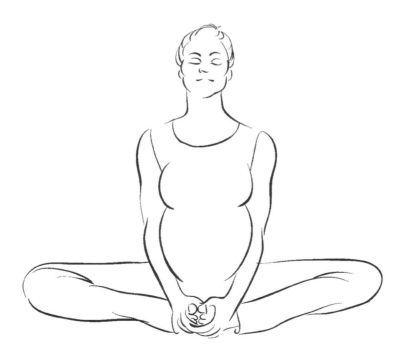

How to do this pose:

- Sit comfortably on a pillow and bring the soles of your feet together.

- Let your knees drop out to the side.

- Sit up tall and release the shoulders.

- Breathe deep and press the feet into each other as you relax the legs.

IT'S YOGA BIRTH TIME!

Active Labor Stage

When your labor starts to feel harder and the contractions are stronger and closer together, you are probably in "good" labor, or active labor. You have to remember that active labor comes with the challenge of fatigue, as contractions are closer together and take a little longer to peak. You may not know where your cervix dilation is and might be curious to find out. You can make a choice here to go to the hospital or, if you have a midwife, she will most likely join you at this point. If you are hoping to manage most of your labor in your home, then you may be hesitant to go to the hospital. Remember: if you are over four centimeters, the nursing staff will admit you, and that might take away your ability to feel freedom in your birth choices.

Sometimes active labor can make you vulnerable to the pain, and just the offer of medication can be tempting. This is a huge consideration when deciding when to go to the hospital, As thy will definitely offer you an epidural. You still have one more phase to get to before you go into pushing stage. You and your partner should have a conversation in the weeks before labor begins as to how long you feel comfortable staying home. Some couples choose to be at home as long as possible and manage to go just before the pushing feeling takes over. Some couples don't want to risk being home that long and decide to use the 5-1-1 rule (contractions 5 minutes apart, lasting 1 minute for 1 hour). This rule does not imply that you would be over four centimeters; it is just a guideline for what might be the right time. If you are hoping to get through labor on your own terms, I often suggest a smaller window of 3-1-1. In most cases, this is reasonable. Keep in mind that you should also consider your emotional state. Sometimes just following your intuition and how you are feeling is your best signal for making a decision.

If you think you are in active labor, use the checklist below to help you identify with how you are feeling and what your next steps are in the YBM.

What's Happening?

Physical Signs

- My contractions are between 3 and 7 minutes apart, lasting 30 to 60 seconds.

- My contractions are more painful, with greater intensity in the peak.

- I may not be able to walk or talk during a contraction.

- This has been going on for more than an hour.

- I am timing the 5-1-1 rule.

- I may feel like using pain medication.

- I may be tired and feeling the onset of fatigue.

Emotional Signs

- I feel anxious or nervous.

- I show emotional signs of frustration as time goes on.

- I may question my ability to birth naturally.

- My pain tolerance may be diminishing.

- I am in a yogini frame of mind entering this stage.

Yoga Birth Method for Active Labor

Concentration/Meditation

- I need to stay in control of my labor.

- My *asanas* help me use gravity to stimulate my baby moving into place.

- While I am in three-part breathing, I visualize my baby moving down the birth canal and dilation moving past four centimeters.

- My intention is my reminder and my promise to myself to keep my labor a wonderful experience.

Breathing Technique

Dirga breathing, also known as three-part breath or elevator breath with longer Om sound. Dirga is the goddess of power and strength. She encompasses female and male energy. Her essence brings women willpower and inner power.

How to: The breath is divided into three sections: the first position is the low belly (on top of or just below the belly button). The second position is the low chest (lower half of the rib cage). The third position is the low throat (just above the top of the sternum). The breath is continuous, inhaled and exhaled through the nose. The inhalation starts in the first position, the low belly; then moves to the second position, the low chest; then to the third position, the low throat. The exhalation starts in the low throat, moves to the low chest, and finishes in the low belly.

Purpose: The three-part breath keeps you focused on the breathing process itself. It keeps the rhythm of breath equal and distracts you from the increase of intensity. Especially as you exhale over the peak of the contraction, you can visualize the baby moving downward with the downward focus of breath.

Yoga Postures

- At this stage it will be difficult to move with a flow of postures. You will use these *asanas* through a contraction to help with discomfort and dilation.

- Use the postures at your own pace and switch *asanas* every few contractions.

- You may start to experience an onset of pressure in the back. Use these poses to help relieve that pressure.

- Support person's assistance is very helpful: pillows, hot/cold therapy, massage techniques, and hands-on assistance in poses.

Active Stage Flow

Using a birthing ball or a chair for assistance can help with comfort in all of these poses. Try to get as comfortable as possible. As you have breaks between contractions, close your eyes and focus on quiet time. Turn off all external stimulation as you surrender to your labor.

Child's Pose

How it helps:

- Releases tension and stress and quiets the mind.

- Turns off external stimulus that provokes negative emotions.

- Allows time to invite awareness of labor.

- Opens the hips and inner thighs, stretches sacrum, prevents back labor.

Comfort measures:

- Use a birthing ball or pillows under the forehead.

- Rest upper body on a birthing ball and rock the hips up and down.

- Apply a hot water bottle or ice pack to the lower back.

- Place pillows under the sit bones.

- Support person can press the space in the sacrum on either side of the spine to release contraction tension (called "sacrum squeeze").

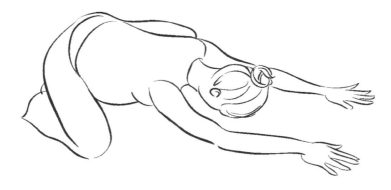

How to do this pose:

- On your knees, touch your big toes together.

- Release your chest and head to the mat.

- Extend your arms outward and breathe deeply.

IT'S YOGA BIRTH TIME!

Cow Pose

How it helps:

- Removes tension throughout the vertebrae.

- Calms the central nervous system.

- Moves breath through the spine and into the contraction.

- Eases back tension.

Comfort measures:

- Rest upper body on a birthing ball and rock the hips up and down.

- Apply a hot water bottle or ice pack to the lower back.

- Support person can press the space in the sacrum on either side of the spine to release contraction tension (called "sacrum squeeze").

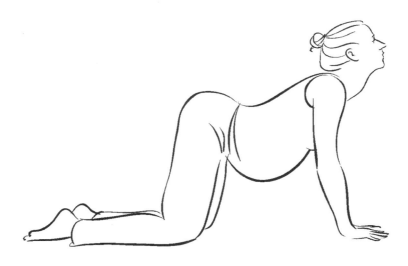

How to do this pose:

- On your hands and knees, breathe in, drop your belly toward the floor, and look up.

- Keep your hips in line with your spine.

- Exhale to neutral spine.

Mountain Pose

How it helps:

- Encourages gravity to bring baby into the birth canal.

- Helps baby maintain anterior vertex position.

- Helps breath move deep into abdomen.

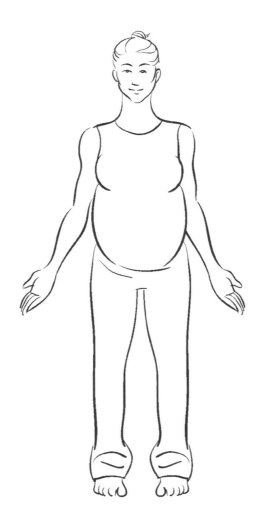

Comfort measures:

- Rock hips from side to side in a circular motion to help cardinal movements.

- Support person can press the space in the sacrum on either side of the spine to release contraction tension (called "sacrum squeeze").

- You and support person can slow dance to ease back tension.

How to do this pose:

- In a standing position, separate your feet slightly wider than hip-distance apart.

- Stand tall and lift your spine upward.

- Relax your shoulders and breathe deeply.

Crescent Lunge

How it helps:

- Encourages baby to align with the birth canal.

- Encourages dilation during contractions.

- Opens the hips and gives baby space for internal rotation.

- Prevents and relieves back labor.

- Prepares hips and adductor muscles for pushing stage.

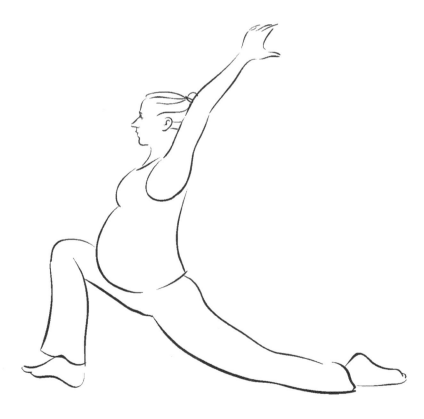

Comfort measures:

- Rest upper body on pillow or birthing ball.

- Support person can press the space in the sacrum on either side of the spine to release contraction tension (called "sacrum squeeze").

- Place pillows under back knee.

How to do this pose:

- On your knees, extend one leg out in front of you, foot flat on the floor, and bend into the leg until the knee reaches 90 degrees.

- Extend the other leg strongly backward.

- Lift the arms up and relax the shoulders.

- As you breathe, keep working into a lunge and focus on opening the chest.

Wide-Angle Forward Bend

How it helps:

- Removes tension throughout the spine, lower back, and inner thighs.

- Increases oxygen to the placenta.

- Opens the sacrum and hips.

- Encourages baby to move into anterior position.

- Eases back labor.

Comfort measures:

- Bend knees to release hamstrings.

- Use a chair, side of a bed, or a wall to raise upper body higher.

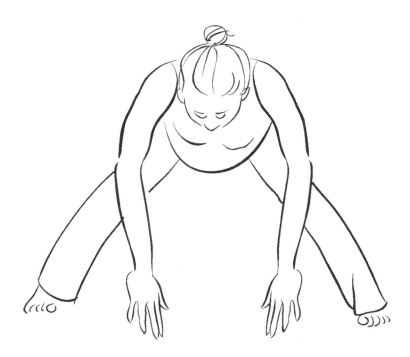

IT'S YOGA BIRTH TIME!

- Using a birthing ball, rock hips in a circular motion to help cardinal movements.

- Support person can press the space in the sacrum on either side of the spine to release contraction tension (called "sacrum squeeze").

- Support person can pull hips up to encourage baby's alignment into the birth canal.

How to do this pose:

- Stand with your legs wider than hip-distance apart.

- Straighten through the legs and extend forward from the hips.

- As you bend forward, try to keep your spine straight.

- Release your hands toward the floor. If you cannot touch the floor, place your hands on your shins or thighs.

- As you breathe, try to extend the spine and straighten the legs.

IT'S YOGA BIRTH TIME!

Frog Pose

How it helps:

- Stretches the perineum.

- Stretches the muscles in the hips.

- Opens the inner thighs and hips.

- Encourages dilation during contractions.

Comfort measures:

- Place pillows under forehead.

- Support person can press the space in the sacrum on either side of the spine to release contraction tension (called "sacrum squeeze").

- Ensure feet are wider apart than knees.

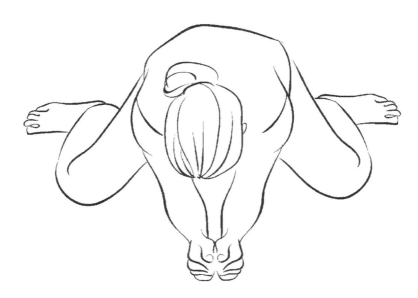

How to do this pose:

- On your hands and knees, move the knees wider than the hips.

- Bend your elbows to the floor.

- Extend the feet out wider than the knees and flex the toes up toward your face.

- Slightly push the tailbone back until you feel a deep stretch in the hips. Do not bounce in and out. Hold the stretch and allow your body to release.

- Breathe deeply.

IT'S YOGA BIRTH TIME!

Transition Stage

It's almost over: you have made it through the first hurdle of discomfort. As you have learned, everyone is different, and everyone labors for different lengths of time before transition happens to them. You may have already had to make some very important decisions that affected your natural pathway. In the next chapter, before I discuss the pushing stage, I will talk to you about the waterfall effect and how some of the medical options can be either obstacles or necessities.

You are very close to your baby being born. If you can manage this last phase, you will have successfully accomplished your desire for natural birth. If you have been faced with making a medical decision, remember you are still on the pathway. Your intentions, your breathing, and your mindful connection to birth is still important. Transition is a very difficult stage physically and emotionally. If you haven't gone to the hospital, now is definitely a time to get going. To be sure you're in transition and to apply the proper YBM techniques, follow the checklist below.

What's Happening?

Physical Signs

- My contractions are coming between 1 and 3 minutes apart, and it seems like there is no break.

- Very strong contractions last 60 to 90 seconds.

- The peak of my contraction is longer and more intense. I can't tell when it is over.

- My water has broken (if hasn't already happened previously).

- I feel like I am having a bowel movement.

- I feel like I have to push even when I am not in a contraction. I know I can't push, though, as it may cause swelling of the cervix and lead to a caesarian.

Emotional Signs

- I am perspiring.

- My legs are having tremors in the thighs.

- I may feel like I have a severe headache.

- I may be experiencing nausea or be
  vomiting all of a sudden.

- I am hot in a contraction and cold when it's done.

- I may be panicky.

- I may be irritable and unable to communicate.

- I may feel disoriented.

Yoga Birth Method for Transition

Concentration/Meditation

- The pain is constant and requires my discipline.

- *Kapalbhati* breath will get me through the
  intensity, and I will be able to remain calm.

- It may seem hard to maintain a calm, meditative
  state, but I can make it through using *pratyahara*, or
  sense withdrawal, to disconnect from the physical
  feeling and connect to my baby being near.

- I am in my yogini rhythm and
  recognize my inner strength.

- *Kapalbhati* gives me energy. My pain converts to energy.

- Baby needs me to work with them here
  as they make the final descent.

Breathing Technique

Kapalbhati breathing, also known as fire breathing

How to: Inhale deeply through both nostrils and
exhale four or five times quickly, with force, through
the mouth. Use that exhalation as a means to find
rhythm with your contraction. You may use a vocal
sound if it feels natural to you. Try to remain in
control of your breathing and not let the exhalations
take over. This will release energy upward and
disengage your connection to your experience.
Keep your energy in a downward flow. Be sure to
take an inhalation; it is key to finding rhythm and
managing anxiety.

In yoga practice, this breath is done with full
abdominal expansion and retraction and is not
recommended for pregnancy. We modify this breath
in labor by eliminating the belly movement and
exaggerating the exhalation. The most important
component to this breathing technique in labor is
monitoring the inhalation. After every three to five
exhalations, you must make sure you take a deep
breath in. This prevents exhaustion and dizziness.

Purpose: This breathing technique maximizes the
breath to move through the intensity of the
contraction. As the contraction feels like it will
never stop, the forceful exhales allow the pain to be
pushed through the body. Transition contractions
are mini peaks at the top, and the continuous
contractions require a stronger breathing pattern.
This is also a cleansing energy breath. You will be

entering the pushing stage soon, and *Kapalbhati* will help rejuvenate you.

Yoga Postures

- At this stage you will not feel like moving between contractions.

- Depending on your freedom or circumstances, you want to maximize gravity.

- Postures will help you get through the feeling of pushing.

- Your support person should encourage position changes and offer motivation.

Transition Stage Flow

Using a birthing ball or a chair and the hospital bed for posture assistance will help with comfort.

Cat Pose

How it helps:

- Removes tension throughout the vertebrae.

- Calms the central nervous system.

- Moves breath through the spine and into the contraction.

- Eases back pressure.

Comfort measures:

- Rest upper body on a birthing ball and roll the hips from side to side.

- Apply a hot water bottle or ice pack to the lower back.

- Support person can press the space in the sacrum on either side of the spine to release contraction tension (called "sacrum squeeze").

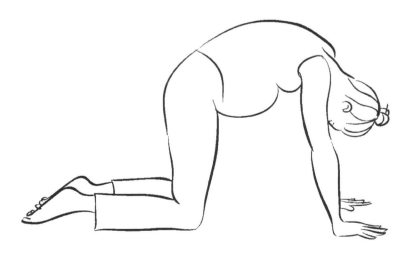

How to do this pose:

- On your hands and knees, assume Table Pose.

- On the inhalation, press into your hands and lift the belly button to your spine.

- Keep your hips in line with your knees.

- Breathe out to a neutral spine.

Cow Pose

How it helps:

- Removes tension throughout the vertebrae.

- Calms the central nervous system.

- Moves breath through the spine and into the contraction.

- Eases back tension.

Comfort measures:

- Rest upper body on a birthing ball and rock the hips up and down.

- Apply a hot water bottle or ice pack to the lower back.

- Support person can press the space in the sacrum on either side of the spine to release contraction tension (called "sacrum squeeze").

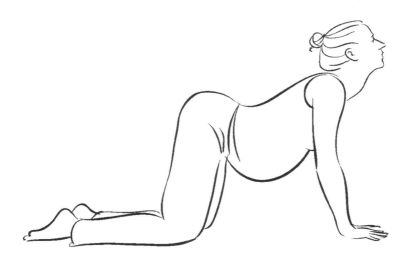

How to do this pose:

- On your hands and knees, breathe in, drop your belly toward the floor, and look up.

- Keep your hips in line with your spine.

- Exhale to neutral spine.

Squat Pose

How it helps:

- Removes tension throughout the spine, shoulders, and neck.

- Increases oxygen to the placenta.

- Opens the sacrum and hips.

- Encourages dilation during contractions.

- Reduces fatigue.

- Eases back tension.

Comfort measures:

- Bend knees to release hamstrings.

- Use a chair or the side of a bed to raise upper body higher.

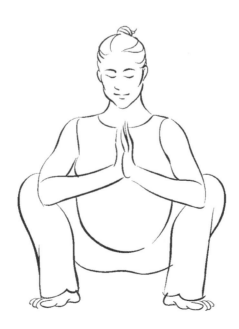

- Support person can assist squat from behind by holding arms.

- Support person can press the space in the sacrum on either side of the spine to release contraction tension (called "sacrum squeeze").

- Support person can pull hips back and stretch spine further.

- Ensure the spine is upright and straight.

How to do this pose:

- Stand with feet hip-distance apart.

- Bend the knees and lower yourself down to the floor.

- Keep the back straight and try not to sink into the hips.

- Support yourself with a birthing ball, wall, or partner if necessary.

- Keep your shoulders relaxed and breathe.

Child's Pose

How it helps:
- Releases tension and stress and quiets the mind.
- Turns off external stimulus that provokes negative emotions.
- Allows time to invite awareness of labor.
- Opens the hips and inner thighs, stretches sacrum, prevents back labor.

Comfort measures:
- Use a birthing ball or pillows under the forehead.
- Rest upper body on a birthing ball and rock the hips up and down.
- Apply a hot water bottle or ice pack to the lower back.
- Place pillows under the sit bones.
- Support person can press the space in the sacrum on either side of the spine to release contraction tension (called "sacrum squeeze").

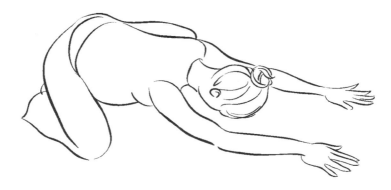

How to do this pose:

- On your knees, touch your big toes together.

- Release your chest and head to the mat.

- Extend your arms outward and breathe deeply.

Delivery Stage

You are ready to have a baby! Once you have reached ten centimeters and are fully effaced, you are ready to begin the next stage, called delivery or pushing. How you push your baby out will be greatly affected by your caregiver's preferences. Usually a low-intervention caregiver such as a midwife will allow you to assume the most comfortable position and use self-directed pushing. Most hospital births are done in a bed from an upright, reclined position using directed pushing, so it's important to know that the positions in the YBM can be modified on the hospital bed too.

In the transition phase, I mentioned that you would begin to feel the urge to push when you have reached the ten-centimeter mark. Pushing is a huge release from pain and feels really good with contractions. Once that urge begins, it is important to ensure your cervix is checked and ready. Pushing before ten centimeters can lead to serious fetal and maternal complications.

Once you have been given the okay to push, you can go ahead and do the work required to bring your baby into the world. In order to feel in control of your birth experience, you should know your pushing options—the position choices and breathing methods available to you. If you leave it in the hands of medical staff, you will inevitably be in the bed, on your back, with everyone yelling "push, push, push," and with a nurse counting to ten. This is called the directed push and can be very stressful. Being on your back can also make pushing a lot harder because the baby must come over the coccyx bone. The most natural way to push would be upright using gravity or on all fours. Again, the positions offered in this stage of labor can be modified on the hospital bed. Hospitals usually have a squat bar attachment that can be placed over the bed so you can sit upright and hang onto it.

One of the downsides to an epidural close to pushing stage is that you would lose your ability to choose how to push, because you would be unable to move. Typically the pushing stage can last up to four hours. Each caregiver has their own set of guidelines before they would consider assistance or C-Section. You should have a conversation with your doctor about their practice for pushing to avoid any interventions within four hours that may not be necessary.

When pushing seems difficult, one method of natural support is to use the mirror push technique. By choosing this method, Mom can ask for a mirror and, as she pushes, she is able to see her cervix opening and baby crowning. When she is able to connect with her pushing visually, it provides a greater incentive to keep pushing and can decrease pushing time.

The Yoga Birth Method uses two positions that are effective for pushing and a breathing technique that allows you to bear down and push naturally. If you are birthing at home, you will have the ability to use these techniques without any medical concern. If you are birthing in the hospital, speak up about your birthing preferences and assert your right to choose how you want to bring your child into the world.

Yoga Birth Method for Delivery

Concentration/Meditation

- I am mindful of sense withdrawal.

- I am aware of the pressure in my rectum
  directed toward effective pushing.

- I am in my yogini rhythm and
  recognize my inner strength.

- *Sukha Purvaka* breathing naturally gives me
  energy to continue pushing as long as I need to.

- Baby needs me to work with them here
  as they are making the final descent.

- As you push down with breath, imagine the breath pushing the baby's feet out through the birth canal.

Breathing Technique

Sukha Purvaka Breath

How to do this pose:

- When the contraction begins, take a long breath in through your nose and hold, bear down, and push.

- Quick breath in through the nose and hold, bear down, and push. Repeat two more times.

- Long exhale, then relax until the next contraction.

- The work here is to gradually increase the hold-and-push duration of each round and also the number of rounds done during each contraction.

Purpose:

- This is an in-and-out hold breath that is modified for contractions. Work this breath with each and every contraction. Maximizing the use of your breath with the length of the contraction makes pushing time shorter. If you exhale in an upward energy or out through the nose instead of bearing down, the pushing will be ineffective. You must hold the breath and push it down to the baby's feet.

Yoga Postures

- At this stage you will not feel like moving between contractions.

- Depending on your freedom or circumstances, you want to maximize gravity.

- Postures will help you get through the feeling of pushing.

- Your support person can offer motivation.

Cat Pose

How it helps:

- Aligns baby with the spine.

- Makes pushing easier on the hips.

Modification:

- Kneel on all fours on the bed.

Comfort measures:

- Rest upper body on a birthing ball and roll the hips from side to side.

- Apply a hot water bottle or ice pack to the lower back.

- Support person can press the space in the sacrum on either side of the spine to release contraction tension (called "sacrum squeeze").

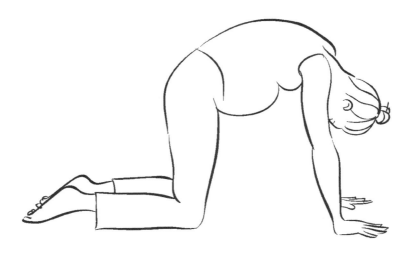

How to do this pose:

- On your hands and knees, assume Table Pose.

- On the inhalation, press into your hands and lift the belly button to your spine.

- Keep your hips in line with your knees.

- Breathe out to a neutral spine.

Squat Pose

How it helps:
- Encourages baby to align with the birth canal.
- Gravity will help with pushing stage.

Modifications:
- Stand with feet on either side of bed and drop bottom part of bed.
- Support person can assist squat from behind by holding arms.
- Use a birthing squat seat if available.
- Use a squat bar over bed (available at hospital).

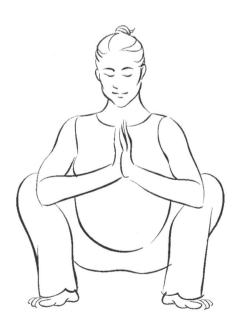

IT'S YOGA BIRTH TIME!

Comfort measures:

- Bend knees to release hamstrings.

- Use a chair or the side of a bed to raise upper body higher.

- Support person can assist squat from behind by holding arms.

- Support person can press the space in the sacrum on either side of the spine to release contraction tension (called "sacrum squeeze").

- Support person can pull hips back and stretch spine further.

- Ensure the spine is upright and straight.

How to do this pose:

- Stand with feet hip-distance apart.

- Bend the knees and lower yourself down to the floor.

- Keep the back straight and try not to sink into the hips.

- Support yourself with a birthing ball, wall, or partner if necessary.

- Keep your shoulders relaxed and breathe.

Once the baby has been delivered, you will feel complete release from any pain that you felt with contractions. You will now have to deliver the placenta. This is an easy process compared to pushing and will be done with the assistance of your doctor. In some hospital procedures, a Pitocin injection is given during the pushing stage. The reason for this injection is to prevent a hemorrhage during placental delivery. The Pitocin increases uterine contractions and can help prevent blood clots from developing. To encourage a natural birth, you may decide to ask your caregiver about their pro- cedures. The doctor will help you deliver the placenta by massaging your uterus and encouraging you to give a few simple pushes. This is the time when you can exercise your options for placenta care after delivery. I highly recommend you take the time to research the following options, as they can provide many upsides to you and your baby's health:

- ✓ **Delayed Cord Cutting** – Gives baby more nutrients and blood volume, increases birth weight
- ✓ **Cord Blood Blanking** – Storing your baby's stem cells
- ✓ **Placenta Encapsulation** – Consuming the placenta raw or into hydrated pill form benefits mother in postnatal recovery

At this point you can begin skin-to-skin breastfeeding. If you used the YBM pathway and managed an unmedicated birth, you will have the freedom to be up and about, shower, and eat. On the other hand, if your birth journey did not go as planned and your experience involved medical intervention, you may be required to wait four hours before getting up from the bed to ensure all medications have effectively worn off. The next chapter will provide you support on incorporating the Yoga Birth Method with medical intervention.

You should now have your baby in your arms. The feeling of holding your child for the first time is indescribable. It represents enlightenment—an unconditional love that will nurture you and your child for the rest of your lives.

Lisa's Birth Story

"Honey, you're at eight centimeters!" my husband reported with pure bliss. I was so happy to hear that but wondered if it really could be true, as it had only been three hours since the last report of three centimeters. I kept calm and used my breathing to get through the next contraction.

I always knew our baby would come early, and he did — at thirty-seven weeks. I spent the two weekends before that finalizing the last-minute details for those who would be covering my work while I was away. We had a routine ultrasound on Monday at thirty-six weeks that found the amniotic fluid to be on the lower side of normal. The risks can be that baby may have a hard time moving in the womb, causing breech (baby does not go head down), and there is a risk that the umbilical cord could wrap around the baby and not float, and in general the fluid is needed to protect the baby. On the flipside, I knew that baby's lungs needed another week of development in the womb.

Since there was no immediate risk, we decided to wait. We followed up with ultrasounds every other day to monitor the baby. That Friday, they said I could get induced if I wanted, but they didn't pressure me to do so. I was so thankful that I had taken the Yoga Birth Method course and was armed with knowledge of the waterfall effect of induction. I was able to talk through all the options and have a better understanding of where we stood. I knew waiting until the following week, when our baby would be at thirty-seven weeks, would make the baby stronger, and the doctors felt comfortable having me come back to be monitored the following Sunday and Tuesday. We figured that when we went on Tuesday they would keep us in the hospital.

A week later, on Tuesday at 4:30 pm, I had them start the induction process with Cervidil. We relaxed with music and waited for the ride to begin. I was hopeful that I wouldn't need any pain meds and get through my labor with movement, breathing, and visualization. I wasn't able to sleep and started to feel stomach cramps — it reminded me of the "Delhi belly" I had upon return from India a few years back. By 4:30 am I was making frequent trips to the bathroom. I remember thinking that I was so thankful again for the YBM course while I was on the toilet and vomiting at the same time, realizing that this was moving things along and a normal part of the birth process instead of not knowing and feeling crappy for feeling this type of sickness during it all. It really helped to know that the vomiting was a good thing.

I sat on a birthing ball for most of the labor (from 3 to 5 am). I asked for the portable monitor so that I could sit on the ball and be mobile and drink fluids myself rather than be on an IV and strapped to a bed, not allowing this labor to progress. In the YBM course we learned how to open up the hips and allow dilatation to progress, and I really think that helped speed up the process. I was at three centimeters at 4:30 am, eight centimeters by 7:30 am, and fully dilated and ready to push by 8:45 am. A half hour of pushing and our sweet baby boy, Shay, was born!

It was a delight to meet him and find out this beautiful, full head of dark hair was our baby boy (we didn't find out the sex until the big day). It was the most amazing experience. I was hoping for a natural childbirth with no epidural or painkillers, and it was easier than I had expected. I couldn't have imagined being stuck in a bed not being able to use my body to help the baby with the delivery — to work together with gravity and help speed up the process. I learned in the course that you can choose to have a positive birth story, and that's what we believed in: no fear, just joyful anticipation for the big day.

7

Making Informed
Decisions

When you anticipate a natural birth, you might assume that it will be easy and progress smoothly. Even if you are doing all the right things, it may not always work out that way. If you are not prepared for what could happen, then dealing with a complicated situation—if it arises—can be devastating for you. In this chapter, we will look at some of the situations that may create obstacles for a natural birth. Rather than explaining the medical terminology in detail, my goal is to bring these situations to light and to show you how the YBM can help you stay focused and able to deal with them effectively. If you would like in-depth education on some of these complications, there are many books that you can read, or speak to your healthcare providers about their experience in dealing with these particular issues.

The purpose of this chapter is to educate you on how to recognize certain complications beforehand and to help you stay present during labor to ensure you don't make a forced decision or a decision that will potentially devastate your perception of childbirth. Hospital births are a safe way to have your child, but nurses and doctors are trained in medical solutions. You should know your right to say no and when natural options are possible.

In some cases, medical intervention can save your child or you from a potential crisis. Other times, medical intervention can actually make the end result worse. According to the World Health Organization, the best outcomes for mothers and babies that end in cesarean section are 5–10 percent of all births—meaning that only 5–10 percent of cesarean births performed are necessary and in the best interest of mother and child. Rates above 15 percent seem to do more harm than good.[1] In the United States, the World Health Organization reported a cesarean rate of 22 percent of all births in 2000 and 31.8 percent in 2007, yet the recommendation for industrialized nations is under 15 percent. In my birthing classes I teach the concept of the waterfall effect. It shows that when medical assistance is used at any given point in labor, certain outcomes almost always prevail. We will look into the waterfall effect here but, most importantly, I want you to have the YBM tools to manage the flow of the waterfall if it becomes a factor in your birth. Awareness of your choices can help prevent disappointment and sadness in your birth outcome.

In chapter 3 I introduced dystocias in labor. These are considered challenges to normal progression, or dysfunctional labor. Each of these challenges can be broken down into specific situations and may encompass one or two issues. Here are some of the challenges we will be covering this chapter:

- induction

- prolonged early phase

- arrest of active labor

These challenges can encompass issues such as maternal distress, fetal complications, uterine inertia, and pain medication.

---

1   See http://www.who.int/healthsystems/topics/financing/healthreport/30C-sectioncosts.pdf.

Induction

One of the first obstacles of labor is whether you will begin labor on your own. Labor is safe for baby anytime after thirty-seven weeks of pregnancy. If you have been scheduled for an induction, it's important for you to know what the reasons are and if it is the best choice for you. Induction is the first medical intervention along the waterfall flow that can cause an unnatural labor. The waterfall flow represents a series of interventions that can happen once one is introduced. It is very similar to a domino effect.

Induction may also be an issue if you have passed the forty-week mark and have not gone into labor. Every healthcare provider will have a practice as to how long they will let you go before induction becomes necessary. This is an important question to ask your doctor. If your cervix is not ready for an induction, then you could end up in a labor that is long and complicated and may require other medical interventions such as pain medication, forceps, vacuum, or cesarean.

One guideline that is used to determine the success of an induction is the Bishop's Score, which identifies the readiness of your cervix for delivery. The softer the cervix or the higher the score, the better chance of a natural delivery.[2]

The Bishop's Score generally follows this scale:

Score	Dilation	Effacement	Station	Position	Consistency
0	closed	0–30%	-3	posterior	firm
1	1-2 cm	40–50%	-2	mid-position	moderately firm
2	3-4 cm	60–70%	-1,0	anterior	soft
3	5+ cm	80+%	+1,+2		

A point is added to the score for each prior vaginal delivery and for preeclampsia. A point is subtracted from the score for postdated

---

2 The Bishop's Score information is from the Amazing Pregnancy website: http://www.amazingpregnancy.com/pregnancy-articles/173.html.

pregnancy, nulliparity (first baby), and premature or prolonged rupture of membranes.

As you can see, the lower the score, the better chance the induction will end up in a cesarean section. The downside to a cesarean section is that a woman is deemed medically to need cesareans with every pregnancy thereafter. A woman considering a natural birth after a cesarean is considered a vaginal birth after cesarean client (a VBAC) and may need to find a doctor that will work with her as a VBAC.

Cesarean Rates:	First-Time Mothers	Women with Past Vaginal Deliveries
scores of 0–3:	45%	7.7%
scores of 4–6:	10%	3.9%
scores of 7–10:	1.4%	

There are many different induction techniques that can be used to start labor. There are pros and cons to each of these techniques. In order to be in control of your birth journey, you should be familiar with these techniques and talk to your healthcare provider about their methods.

Induction Techniques

Breaking the water: A crochet hook is used to make a small hole in the amniotic sac to allow water to leak and encourage contractions.

Pro: If contractions begin, you will not need induction medication and can still manage a natural birth.

Cons: Contractions may not begin, requiring a Pitocin IV. There are risks of other complications such as prolapse of the umbilical cord, failure of baby to descend, or infection—all of which may lead to an immediate cesarean.

Stripping the membranes: Your healthcare provider will do an aggressive pelvic exam to strip the amniotic membrane away from the cervix.

Pro: If contractions begin, you may not need induction medication.

Cons: Usually this procedure is a precursor to ripen the cervix for a gel or Pitocin induction. This procedure can also cause a risk for infection.

Misoprostol tablets: This is a pill that can be taken orally or inserted near the cervix.

Pro: Labor may begin without further medication.

Cons: May not always work and may require further induction techniques. It may also cause rapid labor, which could lead to fetal distress.

Prostaglandin gel or suppositories: This is the insertion of a gel-like substance into the vagina. It may be done on its own or twelve hours before an induction of Pitocin.

Pro: May start labor without further induction procedures. If you will be doing a Pitocin induction, this procedure can help soften the cervix if it is less than three centimeters and there is no effacement.

Cons: This can cause nausea. You may be required to stay at the hospital until active labor begins, and it may require two doses and usually ends in a Pitocin induction. This can also cause distress to the baby if contractions become too rapid or difficult.

Pitocin: The IV administration of a synthetic form of oxytocin, which is the natural hormone your body releases to start uterine contractions.

Pro: This will usually start labor, and the amount of medication administered can be controlled.

Cons: This may cause intense and frequent contractions that last longer. It may also cause distress to the baby. Electronic fetal monitors are also required throughout the entire labor to monitor the baby's heart rate and the intensity of contractions. The medication is usually increased every 15–30 minutes, causing contractions to become more intense and usually unmanageable without an epidural.

One of the first and most important decisions you might have to make in your birth is whether you should be choosing the induction route and which technique is appropriate for you. By understanding how induction changes labor, progression, and contraction intensity, you will be better equipped to use the Yoga Birth Method to manage an induced labor.

Yoga Birth Method for Induction

Your goal is to ensure that induction will start your labor. You want to maximize your efforts and work with your induction method to help bring on good contractions and avoid further medical intervention. Labor will not be a surprise for you, and once you are induced you will be waiting for contractions to become significant enough to be considered good labor. Being in the present moment is very important to ensuring you are capable of managing these induced contractions. They can be more intense than a natural-start labor because they are medically controlled. Your YBM is as follows:

Intention: Be present and aware of your intention; if your labor picks up quickly, it may be harder to resist pain medication. Managing your expectations is important to ensuring you stay on the path.

Breathing: Use *Ujjayi* breathing before induction begins, and stay on that pattern of breathing until contractions intensify. You may need to use *Dirga* breath sooner if the pain seems to be picking up rapidly. Remember your contractions may or may not start based on which induction method you start with; using a calm breath will help you manage the path you are following without losing control or becoming impatient.

Postures: Working your body in positions that will help encourage contractions is beneficial to you and will also get you involved in your induction. Doing the early flow is ideal and allows you to move the entire body. If you would like to focus on getting strong contractions going as quickly as possible, do the following poses:

- Squat
- Mountain (with rocking motion)
- Cat/Cow
- Frog
- Crescent Lunge
- Pigeon

These poses put you in the optimal position to work with gravity and encourage uterine stimulation. As your labor progresses, you can adjust your positions and routine according to the YBM techniques in the previous chapter.

Concentration/Meditation: Work with your induction and not against it. This may not have been your ideal start to labor, but it has become your present situation. Stay positive and trust your ability to continue on a natural path from this point on.

Prolonged Early Phase

Earlier, I explained that true contractions will get stronger, longer, and more frequent. There will also be a change in the cervix due to those contractions. How do you know that the labor pains you are experiencing are normal and not a concern?

Unfortunately, it is very difficult for you to tell if there is a concern with your baby's position or if your cervix is changing. Early labor can be prolonged or slow to start. This poses a challenge, because contractions can still be intense and frequent and go on that way for hours or days, making you exhausted and frustrated. When this occurs it may lead to medical intervention such as induction, pain medication, or cesarean if there appears to be an issue with the cervix or the baby.

There is no specific reason for prolonged early labor. However, from my doula experience, I have seen one of these conditions existing prior to labor beginning:

- Baby is not in birth position—it could be occiput posterior (facing toward mom's belly as opposed to mom's back) or the head is too high in pelvic station or breech. Sometimes a baby may start labor in posterior position but end up turning anterior in the labor process on its own.

- Your cervix is not ready for labor—it is still thick, long, and posterior.

- Your contractions are not consistent—there isn't a regular pattern enabling the cervix to open.

- You are not relaxed.

Yoga Birth Method for Prolonged Early Phase

Intention: Focus on contentment and moderation. Be aware of your emotions and your stress level. If you are having a difficult time waiting for things to get to an active state, you can end up prolonging your labor even more. Your cervix cannot open if your body is not relaxed. Tension restricts blood vessels, which will prevent labor progression.

Breathing: Use *Ujjayi* breathing and stay on that pattern of breathing until there is significant change. A calm breath will help you manage the path you are following without losing control or becoming impatient.

Postures: Work your body in positions that will help encourage regular contractions and open the pelvic muscles. Doing the early flow is ideal and allows you to move the entire body. If you would like to focus on getting strong contractions going as quickly as possible, do the following poses:

- Squat

- Crescent Lunge

- Butterfly

- Wide-Angle Forward Bend

To prevent exhaustion, use support such as partner assistance, a chair, or a birthing ball. If the reason labor is slow to start is because baby is occiput posterior, use these poses to help encourage baby to turn anterior:

- Cat/Cow

- Child's

- Pigeon (lean to side)

- Triangle

If your baby is breech or high in the pelvic station, trying to encourage the baby to make sudden movements may help. Use these poses in rotation:

- Downward Dog (rock hips and bend knees)

- Crescent Lunge

- Mountain (with rocking motion)

These poses will encourage uterine stimulation or help with positioning. Be mindful of your physical practice and don't overdo it. Prolonged early labor can become exhausting, and remember: you still have the active, transition, and delivery stages to get through.

Concentration/Meditation: Stay focused on managing your energy. Relax and allow your body to work through this stage using breath and posture practice. It's important to be mindful of sense withdrawal. Turn off all stimulation and let go of any attachments to an end result.

Arrest of Active Labor

Once your labor gets going and you dilate past the three-centimeter milestone, you then start the active labor phase. Labor should progress a lot more quickly in the active phase, with the average time being between four and eight hours. Going by textbook time isn't always accurate, however, because every woman labors differently. With a second child it is very possible to pass the three-centimeter mark with very mild and sporadic contractions. Active labor is only considered good labor if the contractions are stronger, longer, and closer together and there is change to the cervix as the hours pass. Arrest of active labor is diagnosed differently, depending on your care provider's practice. In most cases, dilating one centimeter every two hours is considered good progression. There may be circumstances in your labor that cause the active phase to slow down and sometimes even to stop.

Arrest or prolonged active labor implies that either your contractions have slowed down or they are less intense; you're finding the pain bearable or easier as opposed to more difficult; or hours have passed and the cervix is unchanged. If this happens, it can lead to medical intervention such as breaking of the water, Pitocin induction, an epidural, or even an emergency cesarean if there is a risk to your baby or you. A suggestion might be offered by your care provider to use one of the interventions, but ultimately it is up to you to determine what is right for you. You have the right to ask about a natural approach to get active labor going again.

The causes of arrest or prolonged active phase are numerous and can be determined by your care provider. Some of the most common active labor dystocias were discussed in chapter 3, including:

- *Uterine inertia:* When there is a problem with contraction timing and strength. The contractions are not strong or long enough to dilate the cervix.

- *Cephalo-pelvic disorder:* The baby's head is bigger than the mother's pelvis, and the baby may not be able to descend through the pelvic structure.

- *Complications with the fetus:* The baby may experience complications prior to the start of labor. Sometimes these complications present themselves during labor. Such complications could be a prolapsed cord (when the umbilical cord descends into the cervix before the baby)—this can be fatal if the baby puts pressure on the cord and cuts off blood and oxygen supply. The baby may be too high in the pelvic station or in an abnormal position.

- There are signs that may occur in labor indicating that baby may not be in vertex anterior position, including if the water broke too early, if the contractions are too close together and then there is a rest period, or if there is a pushing feeling but dilation is not complete.

- *Maternal distress:* If the mother is suffering from anxiety, fear, and exhaustion, this may cause the body to react by contracting muscles and slowing down the process of dilation and effacement.

- *Cervix issues:* The cervix is not effacing completely to 100 percent and still has a rim or lip that won't thin.

- *Medical issues:* Pitocin control was either misdiagnosed or inadequately given; an epidural or other pain medications was given and has slowed labor down; the mother was unable to change positions; the mother is developing a fever or there are possible dehydration issues.

Yoga Birth Method for Arrest of Active Labor

Intention: Focus on nonaggression and discipline. It can be very frustrating when labor has been moving along and then all of a sudden stops progressing normally. Try not to get verbally aggressive or out of control. Before medical intervention becomes an issue, you do have an opportunity to move around and work with your breath and body. Your cervix cannot continue to dilate and efface if you are not relaxed. I have seen situations where an epidural has helped mom to relax so that she can resume labor. I know you are reading this method for a natural birth. Keep in mind that sometimes pain medication can actually be beneficial and you would not be a failure for using it. If maternal distress is a reason that your active labor has slowed, then you may want to consider this route. It would be an appropriate choice, and it would not mean you couldn't manage. Going forward, your intentions would be your most powerful tool to ensure that your attitude remains positive and in control of your birth even if an intervention is used. I am not suggesting that medication is your answer at this point; it just might be presented to you, and it's important to understand your decisions. If you choose an epidural, you would lose your mobility to use the postures, or *asanas*. You may decide to ask for time to try the postures for the prolonged active phase and see if there is any cervical change.

Breathing: Use *Dirga* breathing and stay on that pattern of breathing until there is significant change. A deep three-part breath using *Oms* will help keep the oxygen moving to the placenta and encourage muscles to relax. It will help you to stay calm, present to the moment, and focused on making important decisions.

Postures: Work your body in positions that will help encourage regular contractions and open the pelvic muscles. Doing the early flow is ideal and allows you to move the entire body. If you would like to focus on getting strong contractions going as quickly as possible, do the following poses using partner assistance, a chair, or a birthing ball:

- Squat

- Crescent Lunge

- Frog

- Pigeon

- Warrior II

If the reason is maternal distress, use these poses to help encourage relaxation in your body:

- Cat/Cow

- Child's

- Mountain (slow dance with partner)

- Butterfly

All of these poses encourage uterine stimulation or help with positioning even if the cause of prolonged active phase is unknown.

Concentration/Meditation: Stay focused on managing your birth plan. You may be required to make difficult choices if you are dealing with this setback. Don't let your emotions affect your decision. Trust your knowledge, and allow yourself the time to manage naturally. If medical assistance becomes necessary, then embrace the next stage, which would be delivery.

Pain Medication

It's important to take a look at pain medication as a birth choice. If you decide to use pain medication, you should ask yourself how you will feel emotionally afterward if it was not your goal. If you find that you need medication, then make that decision as you are being mindful of your birth intentions and present to the moment. Wait a few contractions and be sure you are making the right decision without feeling trapped. Labor can be very painful, and if you do not enter it with discipline and committal to the YBM technique, you will most likely require pain medication. Take the time before labor starts to understand the options available to you and the pros and cons to using drugs or an epidural. There can be side effects to your baby even though there is tremendous relief for yourself.

These may be the options available to you for pain medication:

- *Analgesia:* taken orally or injected into the muscle

- *Anesthesia:* epidural or spinal that temporarily blocks all sensation

- *Systemic:* inhaled analgesia

Discuss your options with your care provider. If you are committed to a natural birth and would like to avoid pain medications, then at least you have the knowledge and the resources here to do so.

The hardest part of pain medication is taking it when you tried your best to avoid it. Women who are adamant about a natural birth and end up with an intervention have a difficult time resolving it emotionally. They deem themselves and their labor as failures. This is not the case. There is no way to predict your birth story. You can only prepare for it and be equipped with the power of information to make the right choices for you and your baby each step of the way.

If you find yourself in a situation where you had to have pain medication or your labor ended in a cesarean, then your attitude in dealing with these outcomes is what matters most. I always tell my clients it isn't the birth story that's exciting, it's how you tell that story. Your intentions are your backbone to the best birth possible. How you embrace your energy and manage the power of your mind will reflect how you will experience the birth of your child. Now that you have an understanding of your options, you will not feel forced into making decisions you are not comfortable with during labor.

The Waterfall Effect of Intervention

The waterfall of medical intervention in labor indicates that when you intervene unnecessarily with nature's role, there is a waterfall of effects that occur based on the notion that one thing leads to another. These interventions tend to trickle downward from where you start. As a doula, I use the YBM with my clients to avoid some of the outcomes attached to the waterfall. In most cases, if you are not prepared with what could happen once an intervention is used, then you could end up in the final outcome of assisted delivery with forceps, vacuum, or cesarean section. Knowing the implications of each intervention and using the YBM method is important to staying in control of your birth story. It will also help you make decisions toward managing a natural birth.

The waterfall sequence might go as follows:

- *Induction:* Labor will be forced to start. The pain becomes intolerable and intense, quickly leading to…

- *Analgesic Pain Medication:* Using a painkiller decreases long-term pain tolerance, and when it wears off, it leads to…

- *Anesthesia:* To help manage the long-term pain until delivery stage, leading to…

- *Less Urge to Push:* When the second stage of labor happens, Mom can't feel contractions, leading to…

- *Episiotomy:* An incision is made in the perineum to help baby deliver, which may also lead to…

- *Assisted Delivery:* The need for forceps or vacuum to help deliver baby or possibly…

- *Cesarean Section:* If complications arise, often a cesarean is done to prevent risk to mom and baby.

The cascade of intervention does not have to start at induction. It can happen when pain medication is used; for example:

Victoria was in labor for six hours and felt unable to continue. She was offered Demerol to help with the pain. She didn't understand the outcome and used the Demerol. Two hours later, the Demerol was not sufficient and the new level of contractions seemed worse than before she had used pain medication. This time she was offered an epidural. She decided to take it because she had lost her pain tolerance from using Demerol. An hour after the epidural, Victoria's labor had slowed down, and the doctor decided Pitocin was necessary to get things back on track. Once Pitocin was administered, Victoria could feel some uncomfortable pain and asked to have the epidural increased. Eight hours later, Victoria had reached ten centimeters and was told she could push. She had pushed for three hours and was exhausted. She found pushing to be difficult because she could not feel the contractions to help guide her. She was told that the doctor was going to use a vacuum to help deliver her baby. In addition, the doctor was going to make a small incision to help with vacuum delivery.

In this particular situation, assisted delivery worked with a vacuum. In some cases a woman could end up in cesarean delivery if there is any complication with induction or epidural use such as if the baby's heart rate becomes too high (over 160 bpm) or too low (under 110 bpm) for a prolonged period of time; there is indication of meconium (the baby has had a bowel movement); or the mother is showing signs of high fever (usually indicating an infection). These situations are listed to educate you about possible intervention outcomes, not to imply that if you use any one of the interventions, you will end up in assisted delivery. I would like you to understand the process of intervention and be able to make wise decisions and have informed conversations with your healthcare provider.

Yoga Birthing with an Epidural

Taking an epidural (an administration of anesthesia to the spinal column) might be one of the hardest decisions you have to make in labor if you were planning to manage a medication-free birth. If you feel caught between a rock and a hard spot in labor and choose to have the epidural administered, you still can remain in control of your birth experience.

Epidurals have the stigma of pain-free birthing. When there is no pain, there is nothing to remind you every few minutes of what is happening to your body other than the electronic fetal monitor graph that is printing your contraction intensity. Keep in mind that not all epidurals work effectively; sometimes they provide partial numbing or don't help relieve pain 100 percent. You also don't qualify for an epidural until you are admitted into the hospital, which means there is still a time frame in which you have to manage the pain on your own.

Regardless of the reason for an epidural or when the epidural is taken, you have to deal with your emotions once you receive pain relief. There is hindsight emotion that flows over you once you feel better that makes you think you didn't need the medication or that you could have lasted longer if you tried harder. You have to allow yourself the ability to accept your decision.

Being mindful of contentment and staying connected to your body is very achievable during an epidural, since an epidural may provide you with quiet time and rejuvenation time. Journaling your birth story during this down time can be a great way to stay present and to keep a connection to your baby. If you allow yourself to stay connected, then you can enjoy an enlightened birth experience even when things didn't go your way.

Sarah's Birth Story

My journey with the Yoga Birth Method began in 2010. After completing Dorothy's Yoga Birth Method training, I began teaching Yoga Birth Method classes and workshops myself. I found it truly inspirational and uplifting to receive birth stories from my students—a good number completely natural, both in hospital and at home—who shared how they benefited greatly from using the techniques they had learned in class and how deeply connected they felt to themselves, the birthing process, and their baby. Those who took a different route or found themselves having to make the best choices they could for themselves and their baby still raved at how peaceful their overall experience was and how they felt better equipped to make the best decisions based on their individual situation. They had embraced the Feminine and all the honor it bestowed, and they felt empowered, regardless of their birth story.

I continued teaching Yoga Birth Method classes throughout my pregnancy—to within a week of my due time—modifying my own personal practice to my own personal comfort level. My biggest discomfort was the carpal tunnel symptoms in both wrists; in the third trimester, it was enough to send anyone over the edge and made seemingly simple tasks like holding a glass, writing, or typing nearly impossible, let alone a Downward Dog—but I knew the benefits of the Yoga Birth Method were far greater than the mere physical asana (posture) practice.

And while at first I was disappointed that my physical practice was not quite what I had initially envisioned, I trusted that where I was at was exactly where I was supposed to be and that my experience lacked nothing and, in fact, allowed me to grow as a yoga teacher.

While I modified and often set aside my physical practice entirely, I delved deeply into the other seven steps as I traveled along my prenatal journey. I took the time to contemplate and articulate what intentions I'd hold during my labor and delivery. I faithfully cultivated a meditation and pranayama (breath control) practice that I would draw on regularly to help soothe and tolerate the seemingly constant headaches and migraines in the second trimester, as well as the escalating carpal nerve sensations of the third trimester, which kept me upright and up at night since lying in bed only made it worse.

My due time arrived and passed without worry as I held on to the knowledge that what I was experiencing was a time-honored blessing I was made for and that baby would make his needs known in his own time. As ten days past my due time approached and an ultrasound to check in on baby left some questions as to whether there was adequate fluid surrounding baby, I had already started to gain a growing sense that baby was out of room, and I sensed it was time to give baby a hand. I received an out-patient induction, which involved a membrane sweep and a prostaglandin vaginal insert.

I returned home with labor in progress and continued naturally with my mother as my labor coach. My dining room became my labor room — yoga mat and birthing ball at the ready both there and in the bathroom. My goal was to keep moving to help baby progress, and after a short warm soak in the tub and a shower, I found a modified flowing Cat/Cow and Child's Pose sequence allowed me to turn inward as I surrendered to the experience that was well underway.

With four hours of labor under my belt, I headed to bed with a heating pad — and while I didn't sleep, I was able to rest and use the Ujjayi breath technique, along with meditation and self-hypnosis, to focus on bringing relaxation to my body. My labor progressed rapidly, and while it took me two hours to realize that what I was experiencing was much more than early, active, or even transition, I calmly woke my husband and called the triage nurse. I had just left the hospital less than five hours earlier, and while the triage nurse suggested that I was still in the beginnings of the process, we decided I should head to the hospital so they could check my progression. I believe what had eased this early labor phase was that I had remained on all fours or lying on my side, as *the intensity when upright was quite extreme—in fact, looking back I had actually spent almost three hours at home in the second, or pushing, stage. Now upright and waiting for my husband to get ready, my body was being taken over by intense pushing. I was amazed by the intensity and involuntary involvement of my entire body, and as my husband focused on getting us to the hospital, I remained focused on communicating when each urge came while remaining consciously connected to my breath—moving between Ujjayi breath, the three-part or Dirga breath, and a gentle Kapalbhati breath sequence.*

Within ten minutes we arrived at the hospital, and after signing in I was quickly assessed and moved to a birthing room. As the nurse coached me to resist the urge to push, I focused on using the Kapalbhati breath technique Dorothy had taught for use during the pushing stage. I had arrived at eight centimeters dilated and fully effaced, and as my cervix was completely soft, I was given the green light to push when the urge came.

Within less than thirty minutes of pushing, baby was well crowned but had not fully turned. As the resident and doctor worked to help baby turn, there was growing concern as baby's heart rate was showing clear signs of distress when at rest between contractions. Baby's head was well crowned yet not progressing, so with apprehension I allowed an attempt to use vacuum extraction. With two failed attempts, it was clear our little guy was not going to fit through my bony structure. Knowing he was in distress, at my insistence, I was on my way to an emergency C-section. As I received my spinal, I remained calm and focused on bringing relaxation to my body and to baby, and I surrendered to the situation, knowing that I was doing what was best for my baby. Minutes later, our son arrived not breathing and was whisked away where he would be intubated and given oxygen for thirty minutes before announcing his arrival by attempting to remove the tube.

I was thankful to have had the knowledge of Dorothy's Yoga Birth Method training. Not only did it allow me to manage my labor as naturally as possible, but it gave me the knowledge and understanding I needed to be able to participate fully in the delivery of our child.

Do I feel I had a natural labor and delivery? Yes, I do. I did all the hard work myself, and it was only after baby's increasing distress that I made the choice to give our child the assistance he needed to join us.

Do I feel I could I have pushed back on whether or not I would be induced? Perhaps; yet I had a sense we were already pushing our luck, as in the days leading up to the birth I had began to feel baby's movements at an increasing infrequency.

Do I feel that I lost control of the delivery or experienced any less of an enlightened birth? No. In fact, my doctor told me I had done everything wonderfully and that my body did everything right —baby's head was just too big to fit through my small pelvis.

I am thankful that our little warrior is healthy and strong and that, thanks to Dorothy, I had the tools of the Yoga Birth Method to support my journey to motherhood.

8

Partner Support in Labor

Having support in labor is a personal choice. In most cases your husband or partner will be there for you in your labor as they participate in the birth. Their anticipation is just as heightened as your own, and sometimes partners carry their own worries and fears of birth that are separate from yours. Even though they do not have to birth the baby physically, they worry about whether or not they will be helpful, able to motivate you toward a natural birth, and able to handle seeing you in pain. What if they can't handle the process; will they make you more frustrated than calm? The list goes on and on. This chapter gives your partner hands-on techniques to get involved and help you through your yoga birth.

A birth partner may also be your mother, sister, friend, or doula. Doulas are birth coaches who advocate your birth choices and help you through your labor. My role as a doula is to be hands-on in comfort measures and to support both mom and her partner throughout the labor process. Partners get the most benefit from doulas, because doulas help them with ways to support their partner in labor. If you are considering using a doula, make sure you do your research and find one that fits into your family comfortably. Your doula will be part of your birth experience and your birth story forever, and it's important you and your doula have the same vision and understanding for your birth plan. There are many resources available on the Internet to help you ask the right questions and find the right doula. You can visit my website, www.yogabirthmethod.com, for doulas trained in the YBM technique and for additional doula resources.

Make sure that your partner and support persons participate in your birth plan. In order for you to manage a natural birth, you will need everyone on the same page as your birth beliefs and wishes. As a doula, I find in some cases that I need to talk the birth partner through the pros and cons of an epidural because they are the first to suggest it when they feel you are in too much pain. We often talk about "safe words" that you can use for buying time. I encourage discussing medication *after* a contraction is over, because a natural reaction to pain is to ask for relief while you are in a contraction. When the contraction ends, you are able to regroup and think clearer. If you feel you are losing your ability to cope, your partner can suggest waiting thirty minutes and create time intervals to reassess pain medication. Setting intervals eliminates the frustration of not knowing how much longer things will go and creates shorter time spans to manage your pain threshold.

There are many benefits to having additional support people at your birth; they can:

- offer motivational support and encouragement
- handle phone calls and update friends and family
- help with getting snacks and fluids
- provide physical hands-on support
  so your partner can rest
- be present at your side for comfort
- encourage your partner

One tremendous benefit to having a support person while using the YBM is they can use hands-on techniques for comfort during posture movement. The YBM postures allow you to open hips, encourage dilation, and ease pressure and back tension, among other great benefits. A partner can maximize the benefit of the postures by applying the right amount of assistance and pressure to help you open into a deeper level that feels great on the body and can decrease the level of intensity in each contraction.

These support techniques can also be used during pregnancy. Getting your partner involved in your yoga practice before labor is a great way to bond and give them a hands-on role in participating in your pregnancy. These hands-on techniques will help your body move into deeper stretches without discomfort. You will be able to go beyond your physical limitations and build a deeper connection to your baby well before labor.

There is one very important pressure point in labor that can be done in all these postures. This is called the sacrum squeeze. You will find that the sacrum squeeze is a lifesaver during active and transition stage. It helps to counter-pressure the intensity of the contraction from the front of the abdomen, and it relieves pressure in the groin and lower back. Once you use the sacrum squeeze during contractions, you will find it takes the edge off contractions. Have your partner practice the sacrum squeeze early to ensure they have the right spot when the big day comes. I will give you instructions from Child's Pose, but once you have the spot down pat, then it can be done in any posture.

How to Do the Sacrum Squeeze

- Mom takes Child's Pose.

- Partner, place your hands on her lower back and feel for the tailbone. This triangular space is the sacrum. If you feel around, you will notice a soft, hollow space that surrounds the sacrum.

- Place your hands on her hips as if you are holding a fish bowl and bring your thumbs to this empty space around the triangular bone (sacrum).

- Press the hips together and push down with your thumbs with intensity.

- Keep pressing down without release until the contraction is done.

Hands-On Support Techniques for Early/Active Postures

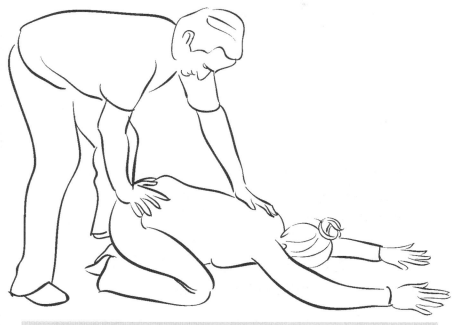

Assisting Child's Pose

- Place your hands on her lower back
  on either side of the spine.

- Press down comfortably.

- Run one hand up the spine and along
  the shoulders to release tension.

Tip: Keep your knees bent and shoulders relaxed.

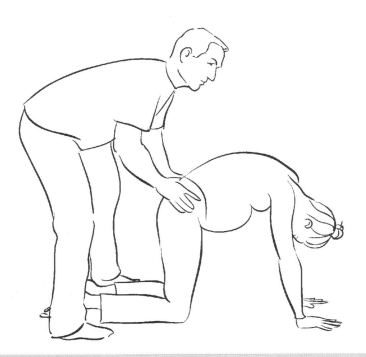

Assisting Cat/Cow Pose

- Place your hands around her hips and squeeze the hips together.

- Use the sacrum squeeze in active/transition labor.

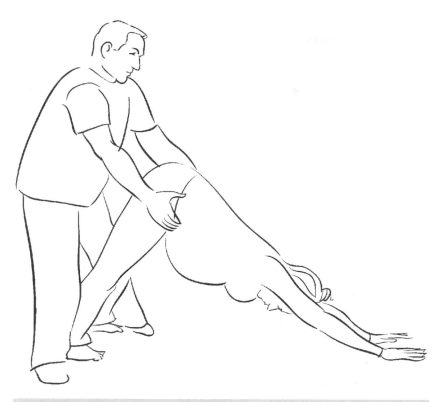

Assisting Downward Dog Pose

- Stand behind Mom and find her hip bones at the joint. This is the place where the legs meet the hips.

- As she stretches, pull back and watch that her spine lengthens and shoulders stretch.

- Keep pulling back as she holds the pose.

Tips: Mom has to keep her hands rooted on the mat and not walk back. She can also bend the knees slightly to help deepen the stretch in the spine. Partner can lean back to make pulling back easier.

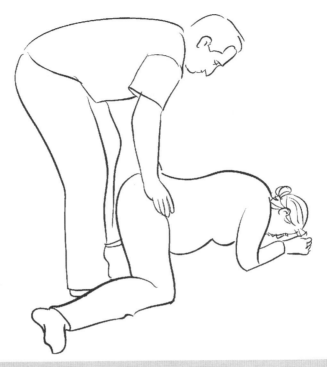

Assisting Frog Pose

- Place your hands on her hips and press the hips together to bring the buttocks closer together.

- Slightly pull back and help her go deeper into the stretch.

Tip: This stretch is very intense. Be sure to work together and communicate how much to pull back. Partner can bend the knees to avoid back pain.

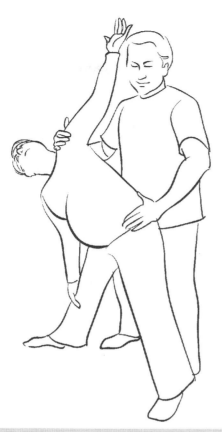

Assisting Triangle Pose

- Stand behind Mom and support her body with your thigh.

- Place your hand on her hip and lightly roll the hip upward toward you.

- Place your other hand on her shoulder and lightly roll her shoulder open.

Tip: Watch the spine lengthen and open slowly to decide how much to pull back. Be sure to support her weight so she feels secure.

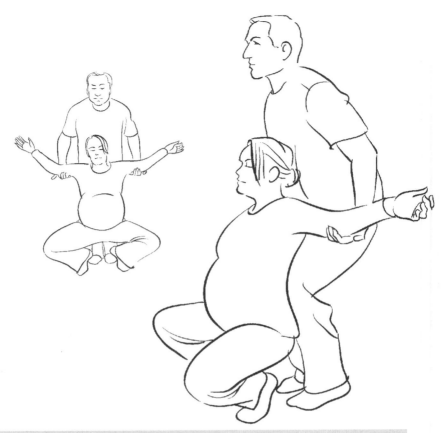

Assisting Squat Pose

There are two different ways to help with squatting. It is important to ensure that the spine stays in line with the hips. You do not want to crouch over and round your upper body over the baby. This will make it difficult for the baby to descend. The upright length in the spine will encourage the baby to align with the birth canal and relieve back pressure in labor.

First Technique

- Stand behind mom and press your knees slightly into her back.

- Allow her to rest her head on you as you support her under the arms.

- Gently help expand her chest to increase oxygen.

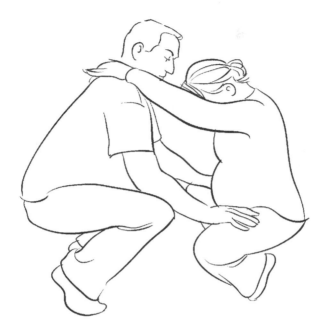

Second Technique

- Squat together.

- Place your hands on her inner thighs and slightly roll them away from each other.

- Make sure her spine is upright and in line with the pelvis.

Tip for both techniques: Sit in a chair or on a birthing ball for comfort as you hold her.

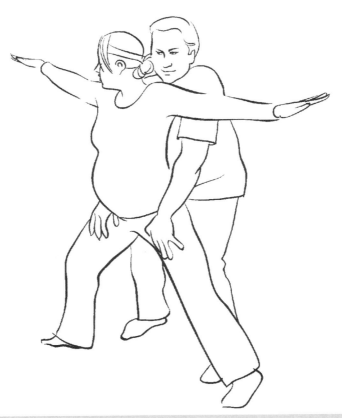

Assisting Warrior II Pose

- Stand behind her and support her body with your thigh.

- Place your hands on her inner thighs, close to her hip joints, and lightly roll the thighs outward at the same time toward you.

Tip: Relax her shoulders by placing your palms on them, and stretch her shoulder blades by gently extending her arms.

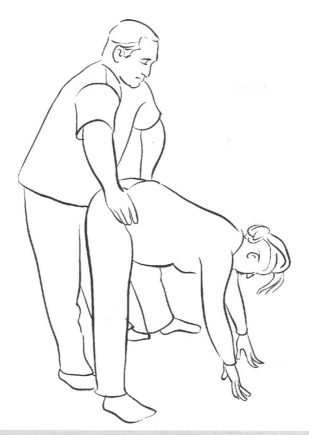

Assisting Wide-Angle Forward Bend

- Place your hands on her hips at the hip joint like you are holding a fish bowl.

- Pull up to lengthen the legs, and use your thumbs to tilt the pelvis forward.

- Use your hand to run along the spine and lift her spine to a straight-back position.

Tip: Bend your knees and keep your shoulders relaxed to avoid discomfort.

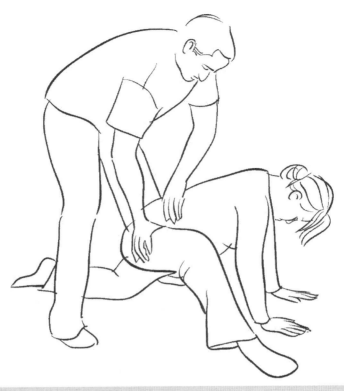

Assisting Crescent Lunge

There are two techniques to assisting Crescent Lunge. One technique creates space in the inner thigh and the other helps relieve back pressure.

First Technique

- Place one hand on her hip and the other on her thigh.
- Roll the thigh outward and away from her belly.
- Use the other hand to lengthen her waist upward.

Tip: Sit on a chair or use a birthing ball.

Second Technique

- Place your hands on her hips as if you are holding a fish bowl.

- Squeeze her hips and bring the buttocks together.

Tip: Bend your knees or sit on a chair.

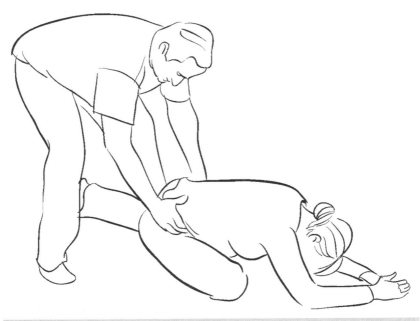

Assisting Pigeon Pose

- First, roll the thigh on the bent knee outward.

- Place your hands on her hips and gently pull back.

- Once you pull back, then squeeze the hips
  and press the buttocks together.

Tip: Keep your knees bent and relax your shoulders.

Support partners, your role is significant. Remember to remind her to breathe and encourage her to be calm and mindful of her intention. If she has chosen to use a mantra, you can repeat the mantra to help her focus and feel good. Make sure you are aware of her birth intentions so you are able to use them as encouraging conversations when needed. You have the ability to help her through a natural birth experience if you trust your ability to be supportive and compassionate.

Danielle's Birth Story

When I woke up at 5:50 am I knew I was in labor. I was cramping and felt excited, but I wondered how long would it be. I started to sterilize the bottles and soothers. I kept feeling the need to sit on the toilet. I did this for about an hour, and the contractions seemed to get closer together. I still had not told my husband I was in labor because I knew he would tell me to go back to bed.

My contractions grew stronger. I wanted to use my yoga birth postures but found I just could not get down on my mat. It was hard to time the contractions because they were so close together, so we decided to call the hospital. The nurse assumed it was false labor because I was not having a break between my contractions. I felt so disappointed, and I was still in a lot of discomfort. My next strategy was a warm bath. In the bath I kept using my breath, and as the pain increased I kept pushing my back into the tub as if I was in Cat Pose. I recalled Dorothy's words in the book that if you bear down you can swell the cervix, so I just kept pushing back and breathing.

Of course, this whole time I thought I was going through false labor, but the pain continued to increase and my breathing started to change. I found I was doing the Dirga breath. My intention for my birth was to be patient and calm, so I just continued breathing and letting things happen.

All of a sudden, I felt as if I was going to have a bowel movement, so I called my husband to come and help me get out of the bathtub. I sat up on my heels and felt the baby drop. Even then I still didn't truly believe I was in labor. At this point I looked down at my legs: they were trembling, and I knew this was a sign that I was in transition. My husband started to press on my sacrum, and I pressed back into his hands — it was such a relief! It was as if we were connected, and at that moment my water broke with so much force. I looked at him and said, "I am in labor."

The contractions picked up strength. I used Cat Pose and Kapalbhati breathing, and he did the sacrum squeeze, which helped so much. At this point the contractions were very close together, and I had a huge urge to bear down. I was thinking I just wanted to stay home. My husband said, "After this next contraction, I need you to stand up and walk out the door. I know you can do it!"

At the hospital, I couldn't fight the urge to push any longer. The resident came in and examined me and told us that the baby was crowning. There wasn't any time to move to a delivery room, so I sat at the end of the bed with the nurse holding one leg and my husband holding the other. I was told it was time to push. Using the Sukha Purvaka breath with the nurse's great direction, I began to push. Four contractions, three pushes each time, and Isabella was born at 11:46 am!

Throughout my whole labor I felt empowered and positive, and I believe it's because I used the Yoga Birth Method. I'm so thankful for it!

9

Preparing Your
Birth Plan

Planning your birth experience is a good way to establish how you would like your labor to happen. Birth plans can help you put those thoughts on paper and give you the ability to share your wishes with your doctor, nurses, and support team. Birth plans outline your birth philosophy on using pain medications, managing medical interventions, and how you would like to experience your surroundings.

There are many different birth plans you can review on the Internet. Your hospital may have a simple plan for you to use that they keep in your file. Some birth plans can be very elaborate, while others are one or two statements that describe your intentions for using medication. Whichever plan you decide to use, you will want to ensure it covers all the topics that are important to you.

I have included a birth plan for you here that I use with my clients. Go through it well before labor begins. You can take this plan with you to the hospital or discuss it with your care provider. It provides you with discussion topics to make choices in your labor easier. It outlines some of the interventions that may occur and allows you to express your knowledge and wishes toward those interventions.

At the same time, the simple birthing statement at the beginning will set the foundation for how you would like to give birth. Keep in mind that things may not go as you planned. Labor is unpredictable, and things can change at any time. Even though you have set out to have a birth that is natural, calm, and enlightened, you have to be mindful toward what is the right thing to do in the moment decisions need to be made.

You will be able to use this book to follow the postures and breathing techniques during each stage of labor. By completing the birth plan below, you are able to incorporate how these techniques will make your birth experience your own. As I said before, it's how you tell your birth story that makes a difference, not the story itself.

How to complete this plan:

1. Read through the entire plan and make sure you are comfortable with it.

2. Write down a statement that indicates your wishes for an ideal natural birth. You can incorporate your desire to use the yoga techniques you have learned.

3. Under the "during labor" section, express your views on taking certain medications. You are planning for a natural birth, but sometimes interventions such as electronic fetal monitors are routine procedures. You can express how you would like them to be used. This will allow the medical staff to understand how you feel about certain procedures.

4. Pain medications are offered by the staff as a way to help you cope. By expressing your thoughts on different medications available to you, it will help the medical staff understand your wishes toward those medications. You may even include a backup plan toward using medications and establish an opinion

on how you would like to experience that stage of labor. You may not have the ability to choose or prevent intervention in pushing stage, but it will help the staff to know which methods you prefer.

5. By completing statements about pushing and delivery techniques, you establish an opinion on how you would like to experience that stage of labor. You may not have the ability to choose or prevent intervention in pushing stage, but it will help the staff to know which methods you prefer.

6. In the postpartum stage you will be experiencing the new journey of motherhood. It is important to ensure that you have resources available to you for breastfeeding support, newborn care, and maternal support.

7. Research your options for placenta care. Many women are now taking the time to understand their rights with placental disposal. One of the major birthing choices women are making today is delayed cord cutting. It is important for you to take the time to understand the pro's for allowing the baby to stay attached to the umbilical cord for 1-3 minutes or as long as 24 hours. There are also services that will pick up your placenta and convert its nutrients into capsules for your in post natal recovery. Cord Blood Banking is another option to store your baby's blood cells in case of a life threatening illness in the future.

Birth Plan for _____
date: _____

My Health History

Number of pregnancies _____

Problems in this pregnancy _____

Allergies _____

Current drugs/medications _____

My Labor Statement

I am mindful of one negative behavior:

_____

I am mindful of one positive intention:

_____

During Labor

My feelings toward induction:

_____

My feelings toward electronic fetal monitoring:

_____

My feelings toward these pain medications:

- Administration of laughing gas _____

- Epidural _____

My feelings toward these assisted delivery techniques:

- Time given to push _____

- Forceps _____

- Vacuum _____

- Cesarean _____

After Delivery

Placenta Care

I have researched these options and would like:

Delayed Cord Clamping_____
Placenta Encapsulation_____
Cord Blood Banking_____

These are my views and requests on the following issues:

- Breast feeding immediately_____

- Giving the baby supplements_____

- Other requests _____

  _____

These are my preferences for my labor and delivery. I
expect that my caregivers and the hospital or birth
center will make every effort to follow this plan;
however, I understand that circumstances may arise
which necessitates changes in the plan. I request
that any changes be discussed with me and/or my
partner. I have discussed this plan with my doula.

Your signature:

_____

Support Person's Signature:

_____

Other Support Person's Signature:

_____

To Write to the Author

If you wish to contact the author or would like more information about this book, please email the author at:

dorothyguerra@me.com

As the author, I appreciate hearing from you and learning of your enjoyment of this book and how it has helped you.

Visit the Website for more information:
Yoga Birth Method Distance Certifications
Yoga Birth Method Certifications in your Area
Find a YBM Practitioner near you
Schedule a Private Birth Class with the Author via Skype

Yogabirthmethod.com

Follow the author on Social Media

Facebook: Yoga Birth Method
IG @yogabirthmethod
IG @Dorothyguerra
You Tube: DorothyGuerra

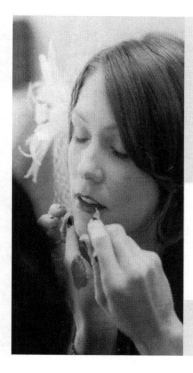

FOTOGRAFIA
BOUTIQUE

Timeless Portraits

T: 905. 338. 3686   info@fotografiaboutique.ca
1525 Cornwall Rd. Unit 1, Oakville, On. L6J 0B2

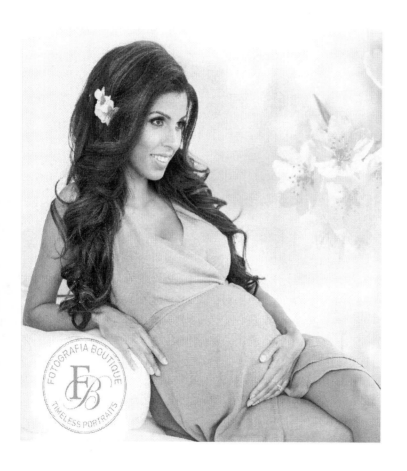

Made in the USA
Columbia, SC
02 March 2019